ASSISTIVE TECHNOLOGY FOR COGNITION

Assistive technology for cognition is technology which can be used to enable, enhance, or extend cognitive function. This book systematically examines how cutting-edge digital technologies can assist the cognitive function of people with cognitive impairments, with the potential to revolutionize rehabilitation. Technologies are reviewed which direct attention, remind, recognize, prompt, and generally guide people through activities of daily living.

Written by experts in neuropsychology and technology development, *Assistive Technology for Cognition* provides a comprehensive overview of the efficacy of technologies to assist people with brain impairments. Based on the list provided by the International Classification of Function, each chapter covers a different cognitive function; namely, attention, memory, affect, perception, executive function, language, numeracy, sequencing, and navigation onto which existing and future assistive technologies for cognition are mapped. This structure provides in-depth research in an accessible way, and will allow practitioners to move from an assessment of cognitive deficits to the prescription of an appropriate assistive technology for cognition. The chapters also make suggestions for future developments.

Assistive Technology for Cognition will be of great interest to clinicians and researchers working in brain injury rehabilitation, technology developers, and also to students in clinical psychology, neuropsychology, and allied health disciplines.

Brian O'Neill is a Consultant in Neuropsychology and Rehabilitation with the Brain Injury Rehabilitation Trust, Glasgow, and Research Fellow at the University of Stirling, UK.

Alex Gillespie is Associate Professor in Social Psychology at the London School of Economics, UK.

Current Issues in Neuropsychology

Series Editor: Jon Evans
University of Glasgow, Glasgow, UK

Current Issues in Neuropsychology is a series of edited books that reflect the state-of-the-art in areas of current and emerging interest in the psychological study of brain damage, behaviour and cognition.

Each volume is tightly focused on a particular topic, with chapters contributed by international experts. The editors of individual volumes are leading figures in their areas and provide an introductory overview of the field.

Each book will reflect an issue, area of uncertainty or controversy, with contributors providing a range of views on the central topic. Examples include the question of whether technology can enhance, support or replace impaired cognition, and how best to understand, assess and manage alcohol related brain damage.

Published titles in the series

Assistive Technology for Cognition
Edited by Brian O'Neill and Alex Gillespie

Alcohol and the Adult Brain
Edited by Jenny Svanberg, Adrienne Withall, Brian Draper and Stephen Bowden

ASSISTIVE TECHNOLOGY FOR COGNITION

A handbook for clinicians and developers

Edited by Brian O'Neill and Alex Gillespie

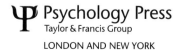

Psychology Press
Taylor & Francis Group

LONDON AND NEW YORK

First published 2015
by Psychology Press
27 Church Road, Hove, East Sussex BN3 2FA

and by Psychology Press
711 Third Avenue, New York, NY 10017

Psychology Press is an imprint of the Taylor & Francis Group, an informa business

British Library Cataloguing in Publication Data
A catalogue record for this book is available from the British Library

Library of Congress Cataloging in Publication Data
   Assistive technology for cognition: a handbook for clinicians and developers/edited by Brian O'Neill, Alex Gillespie. – 1 Edition.
      pages cm. – (Current issues in neuropsychology)
   Includes bibliographical references and index.
   1. Cognition. 2. Neuropsychology. I. O'Neill, Brian (Neuropsychology consultant) editor. II. Gillespie, Alex (Psychologist) editor.
   BF311.A7343 2014
   681'.761–dc23   2014027600

ISBN: 978-1-84872-401-3 (hbk)
ISBN: 978-1-84872-402-0 (pbk)
ISBN: 978-1-315-77910-2 (ebk)

Typeset in Bembo
by Sunrise Setting Ltd, Paignton, UK

Printed and bound in the United States of America by Publishers Graphics, LLC on sustainably sourced paper.

CONTENTS

ILLUSTRATIONS

Figures

Tables

CONTRIBUTORS

Norman Alm, School of Computing, University of Dundee, Dundee, UK

Omar AlZoubi, Carnegie Mellon University in Qatar, Doha, Qatar

Michael von Aster, Center for MR-Research and University Children's Hospital Zürich, Switzerland

Jennifer Boger, Intelligent Assistive Technology and Systems Lab, University of Toronto, Canada; and Toronto Rehabilitation Institute, Toronto, Canada

Pat A. Brown, Department of Rehabilitation Medicine, University of Washington, Seattle, USA

Rafael A. Calvo, University of Sydney, Australia

Bonnie-Kate Dewar, Neuropsychology Services Ltd, London, UK

Jonathan J. Evans, University of Glasgow, UK

Alex Gillespie, London School of Economics, UK

Mark Harniss, Center for Technology and Disability Studies at the University of Washington, Seattle, USA

M. Sazzad Hussain, University of Sydney, Australia

Matthew Jamieson, University of Glasgow, UK

Kurt L. Johnson, Department of Rehabilitation Medicine at the University of Washington, Seattle, USA

Narinder Kapur, Imperial College NHS Trust, London, UK

Tanja Käser, ETH Zürich, Switzerland

Michael Kopelman, Kings College London, UK

Tom Manly, MRC Cognition and Brain Sciences Unit, Cambridge, UK

Oleksandr Maslov, Niilo Mäki Institute, Jyväskylä, Finland

Ugné Maslova, University of Jyväskylä, Finland

Alex Mihailidis, Intelligent Assistive Technology and Systems Lab, University of Toronto, Canada; and Toronto Rehabilitation Institute, Toronto, Canada

Brian O'Neill, Brain Injury Rehabilitation Trust, Glasgow, UK

Pekka Räsänen, Niilo Mäki Institute, Jyväskylä, Finland

Jeremi Sudol, Nantworks, New York, USA

Anna Wilson, University of Canterbury, New Zealand

Barbara A. Wilson, Oliver Zangwill Centre, Ely, UK

Andrew Worthington, Headwise, Birmingham, UK

FOREWORD

Ian H. Robertson

The most famous exemplar of what technology can do to reduce the handicap produced by a brain disorder must surely be Stephen Hawking's speech synthesizer. True, there is a remarkable personality and brain driving the artificial speech, but Hawking manages to be a celebrity scientist engaging with the world at an incredibly high level in spite of the most profound disability.

Hawking's tinny voice has become integrated with his media persona to the extent that it is now an icon of modernity – a token of human ingenuity's triumph over its fragile biological underpinning. This is a good example of the 'neuro-socio-technical' mechanisms by which brain, society, technology – and of course psychology – have come together in the application of technology to brain disorders. The editors of a first edition of this volume on assistive technology for cognition – I am sure there will be many future editions through the decades – have made the first step towards what is likely to be the dominant approach to cognitive disorders over the next 50 years.

The human brain rapidly integrates tools and pointers into its body schema[1] and any semi-addicted user of a smartphone will recognize the psychological amputation which occurs when it is lost. This is good news for the future of assistive technology in the realm of cognitive disorders, but the challenges in this domain are also daunting, as several of the chapters in this book point out.

In particular, many technologies make demands on key cognitive functions such as prospective memory and other executive functions, which may themselves be impaired. The great Russian neuropsychologist, Luria, the pioneer of cognitive rehabilitation, was very pessimistic about the possibility of intrinsic compensatory adjustments leading to therapeutic improvement after damage to the frontal lobes, and he believed that only external prompts and aids to 'scaffold'[2] the behaviour deficits would be likely to be successful.

But Jamieson and Evans are more optimistic in their chapter on executive function, suggesting that, particularly in the case of prospective remembering and goal maintenance, technologies may well improve prospects for at least some of these core cognitive deficits. The NeuroPage system is an excellent exemplar of this, one of the few technologies to have been submitted to randomized trials evaluating relative long-term benefits.[3]

Other types of memory are also beneficiaries of technological advances, as Dewar, Kopelman, Kapur, and Wilson show in their chapter on memory. The use of SenseCam is particularly intriguing and the reality of instantly retrievable storage of images and sounds recorded unobtrusively throughout the waking day offers as yet not fully realized possibilities for some compensation for perhaps the most intractable of all cognitive disorders – amnestic loss.

The prospects for novel neuro-pharmacological treatments for most cognitive disorders look limited for the time being, but the prospects for assistive technologies in mitigating the effects of cognitive disorders, now in their infancy, look very promising. This book makes a great start in documenting their rise.

Notes

1 Maravita, A. and Iriki A. (2004). Tools for the Body (Schema). *Trends in Cognitive Science*, 8: 79–86.
2 Vygotsky, L. S. (1978). *Mind in Society: The Development of Higher Psychological Processes*. Cambridge, MA: Harvard University Press.
3 Wilson, B. A., Emslie, H. C., Quirk, K., and Evans, J. J. (2001). Reducing Everyday Memory and Planning Problems by Means of a Paging System: A Randomised Control Crossover Study. *Journal of Neurology, Neurosurgery and Psychiatry*, 70: 477–82.

ACKNOWLEDGEMENTS

The editors are grateful for the interest, counsel, and support of: Andrew Bateman, Catherine Best, David Conlisk, Flora Cornish, Sara da Silva Ramos, Jon Evans, Michael Fenton, Jessica Fish, Nigel Harris, Lucy Kennedy, Mike Oddy, Frank O'Neill, Jessie Magee, Tom McMillan, Blanca Poveda, Ian Robertson, Giles Yeates, Joseph Zihl, and, of course, the contributing authors.

1

ASSISTIVE TECHNOLOGY FOR COGNITION

Brian O'Neill and Alex Gillespie

This introductory chapter aims to provide an introduction to assistive technology for cognition. It begins with an overview of the long history of augmentation of cognitive functions using technological devices. The chapter will then propose a framework for assistive technology for cognition (ATC) based on the mental functions. The developmental dependence of our cognitive abilities on cognitive technologies throughout the lifespan will be outlined. The loss of cognitive abilities and, thereby, increasing dependence, leads to changes in social relationships and the need for negotiation of roles. Emergent technologies may help reposition individuals with brain impairment within society.

When we refer to ATC we mean technologies which enable, enhance or extend cognitive function when used. We do not mean technology which aims to restore function, that is, cognitive training technology. We do not mean technologies which have awareness of the state of the user but do not feed this back, these are monitoring technologies. We do not mean technologies which perform activities for a person, these are robotic technologies. In ATC, the human user is an autonomous agent using tools to facilitate their own cognition and thereby their independent action and social participation.

A brief history of assistive technology for cognition

The history of human civilization can be written as a history of technology (Mumford, 1934; Clark, 2003; Aunger, 2010; MacGregor, 2010). Technologies are any human-created artifacts that extend human abilities (Kapp, 1877; Lawson, 2010). Bows, catapults, and guns extend our ability to throw objects. Chariots, bicycles, and cars extend the range and velocity of our bipedal mobility. The telegraph, radio, and telephone extend our ability to project the voice over distance. Thus, human culture can be seen to largely comprise technologies which extend human abilities, and, on the other hand, technologies can be seen to mark the major turning points in human history.

McLuhan (1964) refined the conceptualization of technology by observing that technologies were increasingly extending cognitive function. For example, writing, printing, and digitization extend the ability to remember what was heard. Cameras and Google Glass extend our ability to remember and communicate what was seen. Almanacs, indices, and search engine technologies extend the ability to recall information from memory. The range of different technologies, which we often refer to as simply media, have progressively extended our memories and allowed us to communicate them so effectively that they are shared. The key point is that these "cognitive technologies" are not used to act on the world, to do things directly, but they are acting on, and enhancing, human cognitive capacity (Gillespie and Zittoun, 2010).

Arguably, the most longstanding and powerful technology of cognition is language (Vygotsky and Luria, 1994; Mead, 1934). Language makes humans "natural-born cyborgs" (Clark, 2003: 1). Language enables us to leverage the cognition of others to solve problems (Dascal, 2004). But language also changes the way humans think; like any good tool, it makes it more efficient. Young children solve problems better when they are allowed to talk themselves through the task problem (Fernyhough and Fradley, 2005). By using self-talk, including self-questioning and self-arguing, we can enact multi-step behaviors to accomplish complex ends, and remain motivated to continue in the face of adversity to achieve distant outcomes (Larraín and Haye, 2012). Language also enables the encapsulation of cultural knowledge in the form of heuristics, which, again, greatly extend human capacity for learning and action (Gigerenzer and Todd, 1999). Language and heuristics, and other symbolic resources such as narrative structures, are so woven into human psychological processes that it is impossible to completely tease these components apart. Moreover, these ubiquitous cultural technologies are rarely even recognized as technologies, precisely because they are so prevalent (Clark, 2003). They are opaque because we have assimilated these tools as part of ourselves (Cole and Derry, 2005).

Language and heuristics have been amplified in their effect on human cognition by technologies such as writing and numbers. It is likely that writing developed specifically to augment shared human memory, by externalizing and distributing it (Powell, 2012). Its first uses were to store memories for numbers of items, such that two people could later agree on the quantities involved. But later writing also allowed for enhancement of communication and the circulation of ideas, enabling one person, usually a leader, to speak to many. Edicts, pronouncements, and proclamations facilitated larger and more coordinated human collectives (Burke, 2000). Such collective action also required the training of persons in the use of the technology, namely, reading. Tellingly, writing was often less encouraged. This enhanced enhancement was subsequently further extended in power by the printing press, and more recently by the digital revolution (Gillespie, 2010). Historians now increasingly recognize the powerful effects of such technologies in terms of their effect on the cognition of users. The circulation of a perfectly reproduced Bible arguably enabled the Protestant Reformation in which people were encouraged to have their own relation to God via the Bible (Watt, 1994). The printing press allowed nations of people to circulate identical texts and images about themselves and thus to imagine themselves as a collective for the first time; thus, arguably, contributing to the birth of nationalism (Anderson, 1993).

The effect of technologies on cognitive processes has also been documented, with, for example, academic texts and associated thought, becoming increasingly precise and "word processed" in a way which was impossible before word processing (Heim, 1999). Equally, the range of knowledge that people can now access is historically unprecedented, leading to behavioral changes. Where once a medical doctor was consulted as a repository of medical knowledge, patients now increasingly access and read scientific papers relating to their condition (McMullan, 2006). This can empower their position as decision makers in their own healthcare.

The development of electronic computing is a defining advance in human tool use. Initially modeled on human cognitive processes, it is perhaps the tool which resembles us most, has most to offer to our understanding of human cognition (Johnson-Laird, 1988), and which theorists have predicted will increasingly resemble human cognitive processes (Turing, 1950) – and possibly even supersede human cognitive processes (Kurzweil, 2000). Artificial intelligence has become prevalent in most aspects of the contemporary world. Indeed, we use terms such as ubiquitous computing to describe the independent intelligent systems, zero effort technologies that control and coordinate aspects of our environment (Mihailidis *et al.*, 2011). But despite the ubiquity of artificial intelligence, researchers and clinicians have been slow to utilize it explicitly in replacing lost aspects of the intellect; with the first reviews of this topic originating only in the late 1990s (Cole, 1999).

The scope of this book

We hope to have demonstrated that technologies that assist our cognition are normal, ubiquitous, and increasingly integral to human practical and cognitive function. In our recent history, sanitation and health maintaining technologies have proliferated. They have significantly extended our lifespan, which has steadily increased by three months per year for over 160 years (Oeppen and Vaupel, 2002). But this extended lifespan brings with it the increased likelihood of living with infirmity and cognitive decline (Ferri *et al.*, 2005). Medical technologies and techniques mean that we are living longer, but with disabilities following what was once deadly illness. Our chances of surviving damage to the brain have increased steadily over time (Marshall, 2000). Where once inflammation and infection were lethal, now those with brain injury survive with impairments of brain function. The care needs arising from cognitive impairment, secondary to brain injury, and the dementias are prevalent at levels hitherto unseen, and only set to increase in the coming decades. These needs may in part be met by assistive technologies for cognition.

Human societies, enabled by technological advances, have become increasingly complex and, thus, activities of daily living demand increasingly high levels of socialization and cognitive capacity. To have had a prospective memory difficulty before the invention of clocks and time-keeping would, arguably, have been less disabling than the same deficit today. To have had difficulty dividing attention has less of an effect on activity if one has a single task to perform. Our cultural practices are often complex sequences of action requiring high level cognitive skills to achieve. The seemingly simple and near universal social practice of sharing a cup of tea has become a surprisingly cognitively demanding task. Today, to offer a guest a cup of tea demonstrates having an income, being able to use money, interact with shop-keepers, have and use a range of technologies to safely boil the water, and plan and sequence the actions to skillfully make the tea. To be unable to offer a guest a cup of tea marks disability, removes the ability to be hospitable, affects social standing and often marks one out as needing care. Assessment of a person's ability to make a cup of tea, and from that inferring the status of cognitive processes, is a key skill of the occupational therapist (Hannam, 1997). Tea making is a marker for self-care abilities more generally. Accordingly, it is in such daily tasks where advances in technologies for cognition can have the most significant impact. Perhaps new technologies can make the difference between dependency and independence.

Technology for assisting cognition is a huge topic, and, accordingly, we have had to narrow the focus of the book. Specifically, we only consider physical high-tech devices which have been explicitly developed to augment cognitive disability. Thus, we are excluding the many non-physical (i.e. heuristic or semiotic) augmentations of cognition. For example, language (Dascal, 2004), heuristics (Gigerenzer and Todd, 1999), and symbolic resources (Gillespie and Zittoun, 2010) have been found to extend human cognition. Yet, we are leaving these out of consideration because they are difficult to clearly identify, document, and evaluate.

Second, we are excluding from consideration the many "low-tech" physical technologies which extend human cognition. Such devices are commonly used for storing information (notebooks, diaries, and ledgers), calculating large numbers (abacus, pen, and paper), prospective prompting (diaries, alarm clocks, and notices), and sequencing behavior (recipes and manuals). It would take a separate volume to review these devices, their historical emergence and efficacy. Our focus is specifically on the recent development and upsurge of high-tech devices.

Finally, of the high-tech devices that are used to enhance normal or high-functioning cognition, such as computer software, smartphone apps and the alarms, reminders, and prompters used routinely by the population, we will include only those with an evidence base in the alleviation of cognitive deficits. This is the area in which there has been most rapid growth and where new technologies can have the most significant benefits (LoPresti et al., 2004; Gillespie et al., 2012).

Conceptualizing ATC in terms of cognitive function

Despite a surge of interest and research in assistive technologies for cognition, a psychological conceptualization has been lacking. Existing reviews have been organized in terms of the type of assistive technology used (LoPresti et al., 2004), their efficacy (de Joode et al., 2010) and their rehabilitation aims (Cole, 1999), or user groups, such as older adults (Pollack, 2005) or people with dementia (Bharucha et al., 2009).

While extremely important contributions, the underpinning conceptualizations make it difficult to recognize two important factors: first, that similar cognitive deficits arise in different user groups, and, second, that a single technology might be used to support a variety of cognitive functions. We hasten to add that the excellent paper by LoPresti *et al.* (2004) not only coined the phrase "assistive technology for cognition" but also began to define ATC from a neuropsychological point of view. We view our efforts as an expansion of their work (Gillespie *et al.*, 2012).

We propose to use specific mental abilities as a framework for understanding ATC. Specific mental abilities are modular; subject to focal assessments and rehabilitation interventions. Throughout this book it will be shown how these specific cognitive abilities can be selectively augmented by ATC.

Mental functions are specific and seem to have a modular organization. From the 1850s onwards, neurologists and psychologists have produced a literature of careful behavioral descriptions of survivors of specific brain lesions. These accounts began to demonstrate that people can lose specific functions such as the inhibitory control of behavior (Harlow, 1868), language production (Broca, 1861), language comprehension (Wernicke, 1874/1969), face perception (Bodamer, 1947, cited in Ellis and Florence, 1990), episodic memory (Scoville and Milner, 1957), color perception (Pearlman *et al.*, 1979), and semantic memory (Warrington and Shallice, 1984), to name but a few. Thus, neuropsychology began to slowly develop a picture of the functional specificity of brain areas. Later, dissociation studies demonstrated experimentally that people with and without specific damage to a brain circuit differed in yet further mental abilities. The revolutionary functional brain imaging technologies of the 1980s and 1990s largely supported the hypothesis that the mind is modular. We saw demonstrations of specific neural activations underpinning motion perception (Zihl *et al.*, 1983), attention (Posner and Petersen, 1990), calculation (Stanescu-Cosson *et al.*, 2000), and executive functions such as remembering to enact an intention (Burgess *et al.*, 2011). Fodor (1983) extended the case for cognitive modularity by arguing that modularity of function makes evolutionary sense, because it is easier to debug or improve a complex function if it can be differentiated and changed without change to other simultaneously evolving but encapsulated systems. Equally, we suggest, technologies in support of the cognitive functions would be best debugged or improved if they were specific in their function.

The specific mental functions already have a literature on their specific rehabilitation (Halligan *et al.*, 2003; Scottish Intercollegiate Guidelines Network, 2013) and are readily measured with current psychometrics (Lezak *et al.*, 2004; Strauss *et al.*, 2006). Accordingly, conceptualizing ATC in terms of cognitive function will facilitate prescription of ATC. Indeed, it is our aim that the current book will enable clinicians to progress directly from assessment of cognitive deficit to identifying potentially effective ATC.

There have been many attempts to categorize the modules that compose the mind. A consensus statement was required and the present book uses the International Classification of Function (ICF) as our classification of cognition and function (Üstün *et al.*, 2003; World Health Organization, 2002). Using the ICF as a framework to review, assess, and explore the potential of ATC has many benefits.

The ICF is used to define health and disability at both individual and population levels and it has been endorsed by all 191 World Health Organization (WHO) member states. The ICF categorizes body functions, body structures, activities and participation, and environmental factors underlying disability and health. The ICF is distinctive because it focuses on functions rather than aetiology or diagnosis. Focusing on function, instead of clinical populations, encourages a shift towards "design for all," and encourages clinicians to take ATC developed for one clinical population and apply them to a new population. This prescription would be indicated in terms of the functional deficit described. Conceptualizing, evaluating, and prescribing ATC based on the ICF has often been called for (Bauer *et al.*, 2011; Scherer, 2005; Steel *et al.*, 2010). Scherer (2005: 738) stated that not using the ICF in this way "is unfortunate because a common language and structure within which to convey a shared understanding would be of tremendous benefit to the international community of assistive technology researchers, practitioners, and users." Thus, our aim in the present volume is to use the existing framework to support this aim of a common language for the understanding, development, and use of ATC.

This book documents our collective nascent attempts to provide support for specific cognitive deficits. Thus, while many of the mental functions have received development and clinical trial (i.e. prospective memory and attention), others have not. The structure of the ICF allows us to indicate the cognitive functions that have sufficient clinical evidence to inform those prescribing or using technology. The ICF structure also enables us to indicate those functions requiring the collaboration of neuroscientists and technologists to develop future supports.

The ICF conceptualizes the mental functions within the body functions. Within mental functions, the ICF specifies seven global (Table 1.1) and eleven specific (Table 1.2) cognitive functions.

While our initial aim was to dedicate a chapter to each of the global and specific cognitive functions, this was not sensible for two reasons. First, some of the global

TABLE 1.1 Global cognitive functions in the International Classification of Function

Code	Name	Description
B110	Consciousness functions	General mental functions of the state of awareness and alertness, including the clarity and continuity of the wakeful state
B114	Orientation functions	General mental functions of knowing and ascertaining one's relation to self, to others, to time and to one's surroundings
B117	Intellectual functions	General mental functions, required to understand and constructively integrate the various mental functions, including all cognitive functions and their development over the lifespan

TABLE 1.1 (Continued)

Code	Name	Description
B122	Global psychosocial functions	General mental functions, as they develop over the lifespan, required to understand and constructively integrate the mental functions that lead to the formation of the interpersonal skills needed to establish reciprocal social interactions, in terms of both meaning and purpose
B126	Temperament and personality functions	General mental functions of constitutional disposition of the individual to react in a particular way to situations, including the set of mental characteristics that makes the individual distinct from others
B130	Energy and drive functions	General mental functions of physiological and psychological mechanisms that cause the individual to move towards satisfying specific needs and general goals in a persistent manner
B134	Sleep functions	General mental functions of periodic, reversible and selective physical and mental disengagement from one's immediate environment accompanied by characteristic physiological changes

TABLE 1.2 Specific cognitive functions in the International Classification of Function

Code	Name	Description
b140	Attention functions	Specific mental functions of focusing on an external stimulus or internal experience for the required period of time
b144	Memory functions	Specific mental functions of registering and storing information and retrieving it as needed
b147	Psychomotor functions	Specific mental functions of control over both motor and psychological events at the body level
b152	Emotional functions	Specific mental functions related to the feeling and affective components of the processes of the mind
b156	Perceptual functions	Specific mental functions of recognizing and interpreting sensory stimuli
b160	Thought functions	Specific mental functions related to the ideational component of the mind

(Continued)

TABLE 1.2 (Continued)

Code	Name	Description
b164	Higher-level cognitive functions	Specific mental functions especially dependent on the frontal lobes of the brain, including complex goal-directed behaviors such as decision-making, abstract thinking, planning and carrying out plans, mental flexibility, and deciding which behaviors are appropriate under what circumstances; often called executive functions
b167	Mental functions of language	Specific mental functions of recognizing and using signs, symbols and other components of a language
b172	Calculation functions	Specific mental functions of determination, approximation and manipulation of mathematical symbols and processes
b176	Mental function of sequencing complex movements	Specific mental functions of sequencing and coordinating complex, purposeful movements
b180	Experience of self and time functions	Specific mental functions related to the awareness of one's identity, one's body, one's position in the reality of one's environment, and of time

functions (intellectual functions, global psychosocial functions, temperament and personality functions, energy and drive functions) were at a level of description that was too general to facilitate conceptualization of ATC and accordingly they were excluded. There was insufficient literature for a separate chapter on calculation (b172) or thought functions (b160), and accordingly, these two specific functions have been included in a chapter on higher-level cognitive functions (b164) entitled Assistive technology for executive functions. Finally, some of the supports for specific cognitive functions were also seen as supporting aspects of global cognitive function and so are treated together (e.g. Chapter 2). Thus, the links between our chapters and the ICF are as follows:

Chapter 2 *Assistive technology for arousal, alertness[1] and attention[2]* ([1]B110, [2]b140)
Chapter 3 *Assistive technology for memory* (b144)
Chapter 4 *Affect-aware assistive technologies* (b152)
Chapter 5 *Assistive technology for disorders of visual perception* (b156)
Chapter 6 *Assistive technology for executive functions* (Higher Cognitive Functions; b164)
Chapter 7 *Cognitive support for language and social interaction*
Chapter 8 *Assistive technology for supporting learning numeracy* (b172)
Chapter 9 *Assistive technology for psychomotor functioning[1] and sequencing complex movements[2]* ([1]b147, [2]b176)
Chapter 10 *Cognitive technologies for wayfinding* (subsuming aspects of orientation[1] and experience of self and time[2] ([1]b114, [2]b180).

Towards a neuro-socio-technical model of ATC function

Human cognition is grounded in the neural architecture of the human brain. At the risk of simplification, we can say that the brain receives inputs through the perceptual organs, processes the information, and outputs actions through muscle activation. The modularity that we have argued for above is an attempt to differentiate the ways in which the brain processes this information and regulates the resultant output. But when one focuses on the process, it becomes apparent that a full understanding of human cognition, as it occurs in the practices of daily living, cannot be understood without considering elements beyond the brain itself. The social and technical worlds need to be considered too.

Consider, for example, Norman and Shallice's (1980) celebrated model of executive function. Executive functions begin with environmental triggers, which mobilize scripts and lead to action on the environment, at the same time as this whole process, including the consequences of the action, is regulated and monitored by a supervisory attentional system. Turning to the environment, it is clear that it is not a random configuration. Rather, the environment is structured by other people and ourselves, in order to trigger certain scripts and reactions. Representations, in short, are not just in the neural architecture of the human brain, but also in the environment (Norman, 2002). Technologies, artifacts of other humans in our social worlds, embody certain representations, affording certain actions (Gibson, 1979) and extending certain human functions. A chair, in this sense, encodes "sitting." The behavior of sitting in a chair is underpinned by neural activations, training by others, and affordances of the chair. Bateson (1972: 465) argued for a distributed conception of the process of cognition in the world as follows:

> Suppose I am a blind man, and I use a stick. I go tap, tap, tap. Where do I start? Is my mental system bounded at the handle of the stick? Is it bounded by my skin? Does it start halfway up the stick? Does it start at the tip of the stick? But these are nonsense questions [...] The way to delineate the system is to draw the limiting line in such a way that you do not cut any of these pathways in ways which leave things inexplicable. If what you are trying to explain is a given piece of behavior, such as the locomotion of the blind man, then, for this purpose, you will need the street, the stick, the man; the street, the stick and so on, round and round.

Bateson (1972: 465) argued that human cognition and behavior had to be understood in terms of "total circuits." To focus on the brain, the stick or the environment would be to fail to see the functional properties of the whole loop, or set of inter-relations (a point which goes back to Dewey, 1896). Obviously, this does not mean that there is no difference between the brain and the stick, or that the brain is not necessary. In so far as these are components of a functional loop, they are both necessary and neither is sufficient.

All ATC must be part of such a total circuit. Neither neuro- nor socio- nor technical levels of explanation can describe the support allowed in isolation. If someone uses a smartphone to remember an appointment, then, at a functional level (not at a biological level), we can say that the smartphone is part of their memory process.

All technologies require cognitive processing and most require some training. Their use must be supported by the social milieu for the time necessary to allow the functional synergy of the person and device to emerge. The idea of total circuits can be used to analyze disruptions in activity, to locate blockages in the loop, and to speculate about augmentations of the loop so as to enable the activity to continue. More specifically, the total circuit model can be used to systematically map cognitive functions to activities and technologies. The aim is to have a seamless interaction with the world, with zero effort technologies (Mihailidis *et al.*, 2011), where cognition and device work together in a manner as effortless as man and stick.

There is evidence to suggest that functional loops of cognition are not only distributed between neural structure and human technologies, but also between people (see Alm, Chapter 7 of this volume). This is apparent across the lifespan. The social distribution of cognition is evident in the parent–child relationship, where parents "scaffold" the cognitive function of the child, guiding the child through problems (Berk and Winsler, 1995). The problem is solved neither by the child nor by the parent, but by the child with parent as assistant for cognition. Other studies in distributed cognition have shown how people often distribute memories (Wegner *et al.*, 1991). In studies by Johansson *et al.* (2005), elderly couples were found to have clear domains of responsibility for what to remember, so that each would not have to remember where everything is. If there is cognitive deterioration in such a couple it is common for the more able partner to provide selective cognitive support for the less able partner. Functional ability is maintained by the subtle adaptation of one assisting the cognition of the other.

Accordingly, we arrive at a "neuro-socio-technical" model, with cognition distributed in a functional loop, which includes the brain, other people, and technologies. The brain is shaped by others who share ideas, heuristics and technologies to help us meet our basic needs. This model is compatible with the widely used person-other-object models in developmental and social psychology (Zittoun *et al.*, 2007). Human culture has refined the neuro-socio-technical loop, producing a technical environment to support cognition and social practices that support cognition. That technical environment now includes portable electronic devices which can closely emulate brain functions. Equally, much human socialization is about adapting the neural structure of the individual to both the tools in the environment and the modes of social interaction. Accordingly, this functional loop is very difficult to decompose, and it makes little sense to ask which component is the most important. Like each wheel on a bicycle, necessary but insufficient for the function alone.

The benefit of conceptualizing ATC within a "neuro-socio-technical" loop is that it provides a model of functional compensation. As one component of the loop fails, another component can compensate. Baltes (1997) has accumulated much evidence to show that heuristics and technologies can compensate for declining cognitive ability. Equally, there is evidence to show that caregivers can also compensate for declining cognitive ability (Johansson *et al.*, 2005; Stone, 1998). We add to that the evidence that particular new technologies can compensate for the decline of cognitive ability through injury or illness. Recognizing the functional "neuro–socio-technical" loop is crucial for being able to develop interventions which augment declining and lost mental abilities.

It has long been recognized that there will be resistance to the idea of supporting and extending cognition with technologies (LoPresti *et al.*, 2004); specifically that compensatory supports will reduce the chance of development or restoration of the mental function. Such criticisms have historical precedents as the majority of major technological innovations seem to produce both utopian and dystopian fantasies in equal measure (Bauer, 2014). Indeed, Thoth, the Egyptian god credited with the invention of writing for the advancement of wisdom and memory, was admonished by King Thamus not to share this art as it would produce forgetfulness, impair the memory abilities of those who would use it and produce an inferior wisdom to that of teaching by a master (Hackforth, 1972). More recently, electronic calculators led to similar controversy with some finding that calculator use encouraged mathematical skill acquisition (Bell *et al.*, 1978) and others opining that they erode the mathematical abilities of students (Bing and Redish, 2007). Our position on such debates is an emphasis on the fact that humans have always made their own technologies to extend their abilities. Thus, it is important that any concerns are voiced, so that they can be taken into account in future iterations of any given technology. Accordingly, the present volume aims to be neither utopian nor dystopian, but to review and explore systematically the current and future potentials of ATC.

Decline or loss of cognitive abilities and, thereby, increasing dependence, leads to changes in social relationships and the need for negotiation of new roles. Most of us hope to do our own thing, in our own way, in our own homes, for as long as possible. But alteration of our mental functions through neurodegenerative processes and injuries is both the most likely obstacle to that goal and the most likely cause of necessitating care. When we can no longer function independently with safety, we are urged by well-meaning others to live as cared-for, and thereby reduce the risks to ourselves and to others. Specific supports for the impaired functions serve to reposition us from care-receivers to assisted thinkers and doers. As our review of ATC above aimed to demonstrate, such a close integration of technology with cognition and everyday function is not peculiar, rather it is simply a refinement of what is already the case.

Humans are unique in the extent of care and support we show for the ill and impaired among us. Technologies hold out great hope of not just supporting those with injury but extending and restoring the lost abilities. We live in the information age. We believe it is time to usher in an era of ATC, so that those of us who have succumbed to injury can compensate for it and return to participation in our social world.

References

Anderson, B. (1993). *Imagined Communities: Reflections on the Origin and Spread of Nationalism.* London, UK: Verso.

Aunger, R. (2010). Types of Technology. *Technological Forecasting and Social Change,* 77(5): 762–82.

Baltes, P. B. (1997). On the Incomplete Architecture of Human Ontogeny. Selection, Optimization and Compensation as Foundation of Developmental Theory. *The American Psychologist*, 52(4): 366–80.

Bateson, G. (1972). *Steps to an Ecology of Mind*. New York, NY: Ballantine Books.

Bauer, M. (2014). *Atoms, Bytes and Genes: Public Resistance and Socio-Technical Responses*. New York, NY: Routledge.

Bauer, S. M., Elsaesser, L.-J., and Arthanat, S. (2011). Assistive Technology Device Classification Based Upon the World Health Organization's International Classification of Functioning, Disability and Health (ICF). *Disability & Rehabilitation: Assistive Technology*, 6: 243–59.

Bell, A., Burkhardt, H., McIntosh, A., and Moore, G. (1978). *A Calculator Experiment in Primary School*. Nottingham, UK: Shell Centre for Mathematical Education.

Berk, L. E. and Winsler, A. (1995). *Scaffolding Children's Learning: Vygotsky and Early Childhood Education*. Washington, DC: National Association for the Education of Young Children.

Bharucha, A. J., Anand, V., Forlizzi, J., Dew, M. A., Reynolds III, C. F., Stevens, S., and Wactlar, H. (2009). Intelligent Assistive Technology Applications to Dementia Care: Current Capabilities, Limitations and Future Challenges. *The American Journal of Geriatric Psychiatry*, 17(2): 88.

Bing, T. J. and Redish, E. F. (2007). *Symbolic Manipulators Affect Mathematical Mindsets*. Available at: http://arxiv.org/ftp/arxiv/papers/0712/0712.1187.pdf (accessed 22 May 2013).

Broca, P. (1861). Nouvelle Observation d'Aphémie produite par Une Lésion de la Moitié Postérieure des Deuxième et Troisième Circonvolution Frontales. *Bulletin de la Société Anatomique*, 36: 398–407.

Burgess, P. W., Gonen-Yaacovi, G., and Volle, E. (2011). Functional Neuroimaging Studies of Prospective Memory: What Have We Learnt So Far? *Neuropsychologia*, 49: 2246–57.

Burke, P. (2000). *A Social History of Knowledge: From Gutenberg to Diderot*. Cambridge, UK: Polity.

Clark, A. (2003). *Natural-born Cyborgs: Minds, Technologies, and the Future of Human Intelligence*. Oxford, UK: Oxford University Press.

Cole, E. (1999). Cognitive Prosthetics: An Overview to a Method of Treatment. *NeuroRehabilitation*, 12: 39–51.

Cole, M. and Derry, J. (2005). We Have Met Technology and It Is Us. In R. J. Sternberg and D. Preiss (eds), *Intelligence and Technology: Impact of Tools on the Nature and Development of Human Skills* (pp. 209–227). Mahwah, NJ: Lawrence Erlbaum Associates, Publishers.

Dascal, M. (2004). Language as a Cognitive Technology. In B. Gorayska and J. L. Mey (eds), *Cognition and Technology: Co-existence, Convergence, and Evolution* (pp. 37–62). Amsterdam: John Benjamins.

De Joode, E., van Heugten, C., Verhey, F., and van Boxtel, M. (2010). Efficacy and Usability of Assistive Technology for Patients with Cognitive Deficits: A Systematic Review. *Clinical Rehabilitation*, 24: 701–14.

Dewey, J. (1896). The Reflex Arc Concept in Psychology. *Psychological Review*, 3(July): 357–70.

Ellis, H. D. and Florence, M. (1990). Bodamer's (1947) Paper on Prosopagnosia. *Cognitive Neuropsychology*, 7(2): 81–105.

Fernyhough, C. and Fradley, E. (2005). Private Speech on an Executive Task: Relations with Task Difficulty and Task Performance. *Cognitive Development*, 20(1): 103–20.

Ferri, C. P., Prince, M., Brayne, C., Brodaty, H., Fratiglioni, L., Ganguli, M., Hall, K., Hasegawa, K., Hendrie, H., Huang, Y., Jorm, A., Mathers, C., Menezes, P.R., Rimmer, E., and Scazufca, M. (2005). Global Prevalence of Dementia: A Delphi Consensus Study. *Lancet*, 366(9503): 2112–17.

Fodor, J. A. (1983). *Modularity of Mind: An Essay on Faculty Psychology*. Cambridge, MA: MIT Press.

Gibson, J. J. (1979). *The Ecological Approach to Visual Perception*. Boston, MA: Houghton Mifflin.

Gigerenzer, G. and Todd, P. M. (1999). *Simple Heuristics That Make Us Smart*. Oxford, UK: Oxford University Press.

Gillespie, A. (2010). The Message of the Medium: Distributing Academic Knowledge in the Digital Age. *Europe's Journal of Psychology*, 6(2): 1–6.

Gillespie, A. and Zittoun, T. (2010). Using Resources: Conceptualizing the Mediation and Reflective Use of Tools and Signs. *Culture & Psychology*, 16(1): 37–62.

Gillespie, A., Best, C., and O'Neill, B. (2012). Cognitive Function and Assistive Technology for Cognition: A Systematic Review. *Journal of the International Neuropsychological Society*, 18: 1–19.

Hackforth, R. (1972). *Plato's Phaedrus*. Cambridge, UK: Cambridge University Press.

Halligan, P. W., Kischka, U., and Marshall, J. C. (2003). *Handbook of Clinical Neuropsychology*. Oxford, UK: Oxford University Press.

Hannam, D. (1997). More Than Just a Cup of Tea: Meaning Construction in an Everyday Occupation. *Journal of Occupational Science Australia*, 4(2): 69–74.

Harlow, J. M. (1868). Recovery from the Passage of an Iron Bar Through the Head. *Publications of the Massachusetts Medical Society*, 2: 327–47.

Heim, M. (1999). *Electric Language: A Philosophical Study of Word Processing*. New Haven, CT: Yale University Press.

Johansson, N., Andersson, J., and Rönnberg, J. (2005). Compensating Strategies in Collaborative Remembering in Very Old Couples. *Scandinavian Journal of Psychology*, 46(4): 349–59.

Johnson-Laird, P. N. (1988). *The Computer and the Mind*. Cambridge, MA: Harvard University Press.

Kapp, E. (1877). *Grundlinieneinerphilosophie der Tecknik*. Braunmschwieg, Germany: Westermann.

Kurzweil, R. (2000). *The Age of Spiritual Machines: When Computers Exceed Human Intelligence*. London, UK: Penguin.

Larraín, A. and Haye, A. (2012). The Role of Rhetoric in a Dialogical Approach to Thinking. *Journal for the Theory of Social Behaviour*, 42(2): 220–37.

Lawson, C. (2010). Technology and the Extension of Human Capabilities. *Journal for the Theory of Social Behaviour*, 40(2): 207–23.

Lezak, M. D., Howieson, D. B., and Loring, D. W. (2004). *Neuropsychological Assessment* (4th edn). Oxford, UK: Oxford University Press.

LoPresti, E. F., Mihailidis, A., and Kirsch, N. (2004). Assistive Technology for Cognitive Rehabilitation: State of the Art. *Neuropsychological Rehabilitation*, 14: 5–39.

MacGregor, N. (2010). *A History of the World in 100 Objects*. London, UK: Allen Lane.

McLuhan, M. (1964). *Understanding Media: The Extensions of Man*. London, UK: Ark.

McMullan, M. (2006). Patients Using the Internet to Obtain Health Information: How this Affects the Patient–Health Professional Relationship. *Patient Education and Counseling*, 63(1-2): 24.

Marshall, L. F. (2000). Head Injury: Recent Past, Present, and Future. *Neurosurgery*, 47(3): 546–61.

Mead, G. H. (1934). *Mind, Self and Society from the Standpoint of a Social Behaviorist* (Edited by Charles Morris). Chicago: University of Chicago Press.

Mihailidis, A., Boger, J., Hoey, J., and Jiancaro, T. (2011). *Zero Effort Technologies: Considerations, Challenges and Use in Health, Wellness and Rehabilitation*. Toronto, Canada: Morgan & Claypool Publishers.

Mumford, L. (1934). *Technics and Civilization*. New York, NY: Harcourt, Brace and Company.

Norman, D. A. (2002). *The Design of Everyday Things*. London, UK: Basic Books.

Norman, D. and Shallice, T. (1980). *Attention to Action: Willed and Automatic Control of Behavior. Center for Human Information Processing (Technical Report No. 99)*. San Diego, CA: University of California.

Oeppen, J. and Vaupel, J. W. (2002). Broken Limits to Life Expectancy. *Science*, 296(5570): 1029–31.

Pearlman, A. L., Birch, J., and Meadows, J. C. (1979). Cerebral Color Blindness: An Acquired Defect in Hue Discrimination. *Annals of Neurology*, 5: 253–61.

Pollack, M. E. (2005). Intelligent Technology for an Aging Population. *AI Magazine*, 26(2): 9–24.

Posner, M. and Petersen, S. E. (1990). The Attention System of the Human Brain. *Annual Review of Neuroscience*, 13: 25–42.

Powell, B. B. (2012). *Writing: Theory and History of the Technology of Civilization*. Chichester, UK: Wiley-Blackwell.

Scherer, M. J. (2005). Assessing the Benefits of Using Assistive Technologies and Other Supports for Thinking, Remembering and Learning. *Disability & Rehabilitation*, 27: 731–39.

Scottish Intercollegiate Guidelines Network (2013). *Brain Injury Rehabilitation in Adults*. Edinburgh, UK: Healthcare Improvement Scotland.

Scoville, B. and Milner, B. (1957). Loss of Recent Memory After Bilateral Hippocampal Lesions. *Journal of Neurology Neurosurgery and Psychiatry*, 20(11): 11–21.

Steel, E., Gelderblom, G. J., and Witte, L. (2010). Linking Instruments and Documenting Decisions in Service Delivery Guided by an ICF-Based Tool for Assistive Technology Selection. In K. Miesenberger, J. Klaus, W. Zagler, and A. Karshmer (eds), *Computers Helping People With Special Needs* (Vol. 6179, pp. 537–43). Berlin, Germany: Springer.

Stone, C. A. (1998). The Metaphor of Scaffolding: Its Utility for the Field of Learning Disabilities. *Journal of Learning Disabilities*, 331(4): 344–64.

Stanescu-Cosson, R., Pinel, P., van De Moortele, P. F., Le Bihan, D., Cohen, L., and Dehaene, S. (2000). Understanding Dissociations in Dyscalculia: A Brain Imaging Study of the Impact of Number Size on the Cerebral Networks for Exact and Approximate Calculation. *Brain*, 123(11): 2240–55.

Strauss, E., Sherman, E., and Spreen, O. (2006). *A Compendium of Neuropsychological Tests* (3rd edn). Oxford, UK: Oxford University Press.

Turing, A. (1950). Computing Machinery and Intelligence. *Mind*, 236: 433–60.

Üstün, T. B., Chatterji, S., Bickenbach, J., Kostanjsek, N., and Schneider, M. (2003). The International Classification of Functioning, Disability and Health: A New Tool for Understanding Disability and Health. *Disability & Rehabilitation*, 25(11–12): 565–71.

Vygotsky, L. S. and Luria, A. (1994). Tool and Symbol in Child Development. In R. Van de Veer and J. Valsiner (eds), *The Vygotsky reader* (pp. 99–174). Oxford, UK: Blackwell.

Warrington, E. K. and Shallice, T. (1984). Category Specific Semantic Impairments. *Brain*, 107(3): 829–53.

Watt, T. (1994). *Cheap Print and Popular Piety 1550–1640*. Cambridge, UK: Cambridge University Press.

Wegner, D. M., Erber, R., and Raymond, P. (1991). Transactive Memory in Close Relationships. *Journal of Personality and Social Psychology*, 61(6): 923–29.

Wernicke, C. (1874/1969). The Symptom Complex of Aphasia: A Psychological Study on an Anatomical Basis. In R. S. Cohen and M. W. Wartofsky (eds), *Boston Studies In The Philosophy Of Science* (pp. 34–97). Dordrecht, Holland: D. Reidel Publishing Company.

World Health Organization (2002). *Towards a Common Language for Functioning, Disability and Health (ICF)*. Geneva. Available at: http://www.who.int/classifications/icf/site/beginners/bg.pdf (accessed 17 May 2013).

Zihl, J., von Cramon, D., and Mai, N. (1983). Selective Disturbance of Movement Vision after Bilateral Brain Damage. *Brain*, 106(3): 313–340.

Zittoun, T., Gillespie, A., Cornish, F., and Psaltis, C. (2007). The Metaphor of the Triangle in Theories of Human Development. *Human Development*, 50(4): 208–29.

2

ASSISTIVE TECHNOLOGY FOR AROUSAL, ALERTNESS, AND ATTENTION

Brian O'Neill and Tom Manly

The human brain is a remarkable thing. As you read this, your visual cortex is busy representing every angle, color, edge, and movement at all points in your visual fields, all at once. You are aware of only a tiny fraction of these representations. Why does your brain, capable of such massively parallel processing, apparently discard so much information before the point of consciousness? Being aware of the world is very nice in itself, but it does not get you dinner. To get dinner (or avoid being dinner) you need to *act* – run towards, run away from, or reach for something. You have, at best, four limbs, working in concert towards a common goal. *Attention*, that is *selection*, helps facilitate coherent *action*. We act towards a highlighted object, turning down the potential interference of other objects and actions. As human beings, we also take some pride in not simply reflexively acting on immediate happenings but in wanting things and planning their achievement, sometimes over a prolonged series of steps. Selection is therefore not only determined by what is most immediately salient but also by our intentions – sometimes to make dinner you need to focus your attention on a rather uninteresting saucepan.

There is debate about whether attention is carried out by a series of relatively specialized brain systems or is an emergent property of some more general-purpose capacities. In an example of the former approach, Posner and Petersen (1990) proposed three specialized attention networks. The first, linked to parietal function, mediated spatial orienting of attention. The second, to which the anterior cingulate was particularly important, concerned the enhancement of goal-relevant information and the suppression of goal irrelevant information ("selective attention"). The third network, with a right-frontal lobe focus, was involved in the development and maintenance of an alert "ready-to-respond" state. In this view, these systems were attention specific and separable from perception and output, and, to a degree, from each other.

Posner and Petersen's (1990) paper was published at the dawn of the era of functional imaging (relating changes in cerebral blood flow to task performance).

Over two decades on, one of the most surprising and consistent results from this field has been the extent to which increased activity in a relatively limited set of brain areas has been linked with increased attention demands of *many different sorts*. The co-activation, in tasks demanding attention, of the posterior inferior frontal sulcus, the anterior insula/frontal operculum, the dorsal anterior cingulate, and intra-parietal sulcus have led to its characterization as a "multiple demand" (MD) network (Duncan, 2006). A contrasting "default mode" network is active when people are not engaged in a focused external task, and includes the medial temporal lobe, medial prefrontal cortex, and the medial, lateral, and inferior parietal cortex (Buckner et al., 2008). At first glance, the common recruitment of MD regions across many sorts of tasks appears at odds with the notion of different kinds of attention that can be selectively impaired. This conclusion would be premature, but does prompt a slightly different perspective. It is certainly the case that, in healthy participants, separate attention factors (e.g. selective and sustained attention factors) are detectable, but are generally superimposed upon positive correlations between many different types of attention test (high scorers on one attention test tend to score high on other tests; high scorers on a sustained attention test tend to do particularly well on another sustained attention test, see e.g. Underbjerg et al., 2013). There are similar examples in the clinical literature. For example, patients with unilateral neglect, defined by problems in spatial attention, also tend to have considerable problems with other kinds of attention (e.g. Husain and Rorden, 2003; Robertson et al., 1997b). This is important, as we shall discuss, in thinking about means of improving spatial attention (including via assistive technologies) that do not necessarily focus on the spatial component. The range and spread of cerebral attention regions helps explain why problems with focus are so common after brain injury from strokes, traumas, neoplasms, infections, and dementias, as well as a wide range of developmental and psychiatric conditions (e.g. Spira and Fischel, 2005; Duffner et al., 2000; Sterzi et al., 1993; Parasuraman and Nestor, 1991; Morris et al., 2012; Manly et al., 2004).

Arousal

Arousal can be defined as the state of readiness or reactivity of the body/nervous system to detect and respond to stimuli. Research has highlighted the central importance to arousal of the reticular activating system (RAS), a cellular circuit, arising in the brainstem and electrochemically (via adrenergic and cholinergic projections) increasing cortical activity (in lateral prefrontal and parietal areas), and thereby modulating attentional processing (Steriade, 1996).

Sufficient arousal is a prerequisite for many forms of attention. Every 24 hours we go through a circadian cycle in which, at its depths (sleep), we are relatively unresponsive to external stimuli. Even when awake there is predictable variability; for example, weaker attention early in the morning and late at night (e.g. Manly et al., 2002). Patients in coma (in which there are no sleep–wake cycles) and the vegetative state (in which there are) may appear largely unresponsive to external stimuli. At the other extreme, in an important demonstration that more is not necessarily better when it comes to arousal, Yerkes and Dodson (1908) described an inverted U-shaped function in which low levels of arousal *and* excessive levels of arousal were associated with reduced attention performance. Excessive arousal (e.g. when highly anxious or angry – the "red mist") can impair attention and judgment. Where the peak falls varies according to the task being undertaken. Understanding the effects of insufficient and excessive levels of arousal will be important to conceptualizing our clinical interventions.

Assistive technologies in attention

In the following sections we differentiate between interventions for "spatial" and "non-spatial" attention. By "spatial" we primarily mean interventions for unilateral spatial neglect. By "non-spatial" we mean any other kind of attention problem that is not marked by systematic bias away from one side of space. We will begin with the more general (and more frequently impaired) non-spatial attention and then move to the more specific unilateral neglect.

Strategic manipulation of non-spatial attention

"Every one knows what attention is," wrote William James (1890: 403), referring to our subjective sense of focus, awareness, and limited capacity. Accordingly, we act to enhance and maintain our attention to important activities. We turn down speech radio when writing or telephoning, seek a non-salient gaze point when composing a thought and invite our office mates to move distracting discussions elsewhere as a deadline approaches.

These "interventions" appear so obvious as to require little scientific research. However, there are indications that we may differ in what constitutes optimal conditions. For example, Kallinen and Ravaja (2007) compared the effects of listening to a news broadcast over speakers or headphones (where extraneous sound is reduced). Headphone listening was preferred, and elicited more positive emotional responses and was associated with better attention to the material. However, the reduction in dependence on endogenous attentional processes (with headphones) preferentially benefitted those scoring lower on sociability and activity personality scales. Speaker listening prompted greater physiological arousal as indexed by electrodermal activity and was preferred by high sensation-seeking scorers. Sörqvist (2010) reviewed literature on the effect of task irrelevant sound on cognitive performance and concluded that those with limited capacity working memory are likely to have improved function with noise abatement technologies, including noise cancelling ear plugs. Work with healthy participants produced mixed results as to the costs or benefits of extraneous noise on sustained attention performance (i.e. the noise may both distract from the discriminations required by the task and help you to stay sufficiently alert to perform it (Poulton, 1977)).

Clinically, the following are useful to take into account. Where is the person required to pay attention? Is the person aware of the need to protect limited attentional resources? Behavioral experiments allow co-exploration of factors affecting attention to meaningful activities, such as background music, taking breaks, or working at different times of the day.

Automated manipulation of non-spatial attention

Attention assisting technologies are in general use. Road vehicles are a good example. Primarily, your attention should be on the road with minimal competition from displays. When urgent events require attention, salient flashing indicators and sounds indicate low oil or fuel. Car manufacturers have explored technology to detect behavioral signs of drowsiness and trigger mechanisms to promote alertness. Indeed, self-driving cars appear able to assume all of the attentional demands, potentially assisting many people who are currently prevented from driving.

Randomly timed cues for non-spatial attention

Vehicles can employ attention modifiers easily. Car operation behavior is relatively constrained, the goals of the activity are simply defined ("A to B, safely"), and relevant objects and events can be monitored easily. An inherent challenge in trying to support attention in "free range" human activity is awareness of the person's intention at that moment and to what, of the myriad external and internal events, should attention be paid.

One way around this is not to draw attention to anything specific, but to draw people's attention to the *process* of paying attention. Manly *et al.* (2004) asked participants, including stroke survivors with attention problems, to perform the Sustained Attention to Response Test (SART; Robertson *et al.*, 1997a). In this rather simple measure, single digits are presented on a computer screen at a regular rate of about one per second. The participant's job is to press a single response key for each digit presented, withholding the response on a nominated "no-go" digit. The random order of the digits makes the occurrence of a no-go trial unpredictable. Most people are able to withhold their responses correctly for the many of the 25 no-go trials typically presented. However, the majority of us will take our mind off the goal and produce erroneous responses during the five minutes of the test (in fact, usually about five errors; Manly *et al.*, 2000). These rates are increased following brain injury (Robertson *et al.*, 1997a). Attention wanders from the simple repetitive task, leaving the response hand "unsupervised" and error prone. What would happen if participants were periodically reminded to keep paying attention? Accordingly, a series of tones were presented linked with the instruction, "if you hear a tone, try to think about what you are doing in the test." The resulting performance improved, particularly in the period immediately following a tone. O'Connor *et al.* (2011) examined similar effects in healthy participants undergoing functional magnetic resonance imaging (fMRI). They found that the "pay attention" tones reduced activation in right-frontal regions of the MD network, interpreted as reducing demands on this endogenous attentional system. These results were theoretically interesting because they indicated that attention modulation helped participants inhibit their responses; but were they of practical value? For example, do people habituate to (learn to ignore) the tones on longer trials?

Children with a diagnosis of attention deficit hyperactivity disorder (ADHD) can have problems in maintaining their attention during school activities. Rich (2009) demonstrated performance improvements in three such children when wearing a watch (Watchminder) that issued random "pay attention" vibrations. Manly *et al.* (2004) examined whether random cueing could improve the performance of people with executive problems following brain injury. The patients completed the Hotel Test that required attempting a little of each of six hotel management tasks (e.g. sorting coins, alphabetizing conference labels, etc.) given insufficient time (15 minutes) to complete even one. Good performance requires maintaining the goal, monitoring the passage of time, and activity-switching. Randomly timed tones, previously linked with the instruction "think about what you are doing" significantly improved the patients' performance (to within the range of an IQ-matched neurotypical control group). The result was interesting in confirming that poor performance without the tones was unlikely to be related to poor motivation or incomprehension of the instructions; rather, the content-free cues directed attention to the internal representation of intentions. The question remained, however, whether such effects could usefully persist.

Fish and colleagues (Fish *et al.*, 2007) examined this over a two-week period, again in patients with everyday organizational problems following brain injury. Participants were taught Goal Management Training (Levine *et al.*, 2000) in which the cue word "STOP!" (*S*top, *T*hink, *O*rganize, *P*lan) was linked to review of intentions. They were then tasked to phone the study's answerphone at set times daily. The effect of adding automated cueing to Goal Management Training was assessed by comparing performance on a random seven of fourteen days where participants received (eight) random "STOP" messages (not within 30 minutes of the to-be-made phone calls). On days receiving cues, design-blinded participants were significantly better able to make the calls. The effect of random cues, for participants trained to keep in mind, review, and *execute* their intentions, persisted over at least two weeks.

Biofeedback training for non-spatial attention

Biofeedback is the receipt of real-time information about some physiological marker. Targets have included heart rate, skin sweat levels, brain activity patterns from electroencephalography (EEG), and fMRI. Biofeedback has potential to both train increased and persisting regulation of attention, and as an adjunctive support during activities.

EEG biofeedback training for children diagnosed with ADHD has a large literature, albeit with few rigorously controlled studies. The large study by Monastra and colleagues (Monastra *et al.*, 2002) is an exception with which we represent the area. Their approach was informed by the observation of reduced EEG activity in the 12–15 Hz ("sensory motor rhythm; SMR") or 16–20 Hz ("beta") bands, and increased activity in slower bands (4–8 Hz; "theta") in ADHD children compared with non-ADHD groups. (Stimulant medications such as methylphenidate (Ritalin) can reverse this EEG pattern and produce benefits in attention.) The study examined whether biofeedback of the relative activity in these EEG bands could help ADHD children achieve and maintain similar levels to children without ADHD, and whether this affected performance and behavior. Accordingly, 100 children were allocated to "Comprehensive Clinical Care" (CCC: good quality conventional management comprising medication, parental counseling, and school input) or the same package plus 30–40 minutes weekly EEG feedback training. Reaching target levels of activity within the SMR and beta EEG bands led to visual and auditory feedback and points for later cash rewards. Without specific instruction on techniques to increase attention, EEG fluctuations corresponding to increased attention were shaped by operant conditioning. Children were trained to reach a normative criterion EEG band activity for 40 minutes (which took 17–33 hours of training). At intake, the two groups had similar levels of ADHD symptoms, attention test performance, and EEG indices. After training, the biofeedback group, even without medication, showed relative power in the selected EEG bands (during reading and drawing tasks) in the same range as children without ADHD (something the CCC group only achieved when tested on medication). The biofeedback group also showed greater sustained improvement on teacher and parent ratings and on attention test scores than the CCC group. A review by the same group (Monastra et al., 2005) concluded that EEG biofeedback was "probably efficacious" in treating ADHD, but called for more studies with randomized control. More recently, Arns et al. (2009) reviewed 10 studies of EEG biofeedback in ADHD and reported Cohen's d effect sizes of 1.02 in teacher-rated inattention; 0.71 in hyperactivity and 0.94 in impulsivity ratings (each a large effect). The practicality and acceptability of the training time is questionable, but given the potential side effects of stimulant medication, efficacious attention training technologies should be more available. There have been reports of beneficial EEG arousal training following traumatic brain injury, but future studies require better control (Thatcher, 2000).

EEG requires time to apply scalp electrodes and a good deal of signal processing power. An alternative biomarker of arousal is electrodermal activity. In this paradigm, changes in conductivity between two electrodes on the skin (rapidly reflecting sympathetic nervous system activity) are smoothed and calibrated to produce useable auditory or visual feedback. Greco and colleagues (Greco et al., 2013) examined whether galvanic skin response (GSR) feedback could assist elderly people by increasing their awareness of their current state of arousal and the effects of potential modulators, such as adopting a more upright posture or deep diaphragmatic breathing. A padded "alertness cushion" was developed, with electrodes that attached to the user's fingers and a central biofeedback display. Forty participants (aged 60–83), with self-reported memory difficulties, were randomly assigned to biofeedback-informed self-alerting training or a psychoeducational control (daily over four weeks). The biofeedback condition was associated with improved performance on a measure of executive function (category fluency). The convenient and low-cost intervention was achieved by posting equipment to the participants who self-administered the training.

Cognitive training for attention

The computer games industry, at least in the UK, is reported to generate more revenue than the music and film industries combined. Computer games can present attractive graphics, adapt to the user's performance level, and reinforce persistent performance to produce entertaining and highly immersive experiences. Games can be played in the home, on the bus, and even (we are told) in the workplace, often at little cost. Many attempts are underway to recruit these features in the service of education and "cognitive training" of all sorts. Whilst there is little or no published evidence behind most commercial "brain training" packages, there are exceptions.

Working Memory Training (WMT) is a particularly advanced example. Working memory refers to the retention and manipulation of information over relatively short intervals and is a concept closely interwoven with that of attention (Baddeley, 1993). Working memory tasks, in spatial and verbal domains, are relatively easy to contrive and manipulate in terms of difficulty. Klingberg *et al.* (2005) reported the results of a trial in which 53 children meeting the diagnosis of ADHD were randomly allocated to one of two conditions; approximately 25 x 40 minute home-based sessions of progressive WMT (maintaining challenge by varying the difficulty according to performance) or a similar duration of easy, non-progressive WMT. The progressive training was linked with improved performance not only on the trained tasks, but also on untrained measures of working memory (digit span, spatial span, both forwards and backwards), attention (Stroop test), reasoning (Raven's Colored Progressive Matrices), and parental ratings of ADHD symptoms. The large effect sizes were maintained at 3-month follow-up. There has been replication of the findings (Holmes *et al.*, 2009) and preliminary results indicate effects in adults following stroke (Westerberg *et al.*, 2007). The mechanisms behind these apparently generalized improvements are not yet clearly understood; for example, whether they represent genuine increased WM, or attention capacity or improved strategy development, "stamina," and confidence. Understanding the conditions and mechanisms that foster generalization are important current research aims.

Face-to-face attention training approaches with established efficacy may be deemed to have initial proof-of-concept for a computerized version. Promising candidates would thus include Goal Management Training (e.g. Levine *et al.*, 2007); Problem Solving Therapy (Miotto *et al.*, 2009), and varieties of Mindfulness-based training (Novakovic-Agopian *et al.*, 2011) each of which has elements argued to support the strategic deployment of attention.

Music

From some of the most recent technological developments we now briefly turn to one of the oldest. Up-beat music can raise arousal levels at the time and for an hour or more following exposure (Gaston, 1968). Sedate pieces can lower arousal levels over a similar timeframe. The effect of music can be observed behaviorally; audiences applaud more loudly and sit with a more erect posture after hearing stimulating, compared with sedate, music (Gaston, 1968). The effect may be additive, as sitting with an erect posture also increases the ability to pay attention (Greco *et al.*, 2013).

In a series of four single cases, Wilson *et al.* (1992) examined the immediate effect of music stimulation of patients in persistent vegetative state. In two of the four there were significant behavior changes suggestive of increased arousal. O'Kelly *et al.* (2013) investigated the effect of music therapy on 20 healthy participants and 21 individuals in vegetative and minimally conscious states. They examined the relative effects of preferred music, disliked music, improvised music entrained to respiration, white noise, and silence on participants' behavioral responses, electroencephalogram (EEG) activity, heart rate variability, and respiration. In the healthy cohort, preferred music led to significant increases in respiration rate and globally enhanced EEG power spectra responses, corresponding with increases in arousal and attention. The patients' responses were heterogeneous, but significant EEG amplitude increases and increased blink rate (a behavioral indicator of arousal) were associated with preferred music. This modulatory effect of a brief intervention suggests the study of longer interventions as part of rehabilitation, as well as the music response as a prognostic indicator.

Interventions for spatial attention

Unilateral spatial neglect is a surprisingly common consequence of right (85 percent of acute survivors show signs) and left hemisphere (65 percent) stroke in which awareness of information in contralesional space is impaired (Stone *et al.*, 1993). It offers fascinating insights into the nature of conscious experience. For example, information from neglected space may unconsciously prime behavior, and neglect may manifest across different sensory modalities including mental representations (Bisiach and Luzzatti, 1978). Left neglect is markedly more persistent than right and is linked with poor recovery and outcome (Paolucci *et al.*, 2003).

Spatial neglect is not clear-cut, but rather represents a probabilistic gradient with information on the neglected side more likely to be missed. This is important, because if a patient can *sometimes* search and detect information on the neglected side, it suggests residual function that can be augmented.

Can patients be re-trained to scan to the left? Lawson (1962) worked with a patient who missed leftward words and letters when reading. She was encouraged to scan to the left of the page to find a red margin before reading each line. This led to significant improvements, but these were curiously limited to the trained text. Disappointing generalization to untrained tasks has characterized subsequent visual-scanning techniques; for example, a machine with left sweeping lights (e.g. Diller and Weinberg, 1977; Robertson, 1990). Pizzamiglio and colleagues (e.g. Antonucci *et al.*, 1995) described a (40 hour) program in which patients were cued to make leftward visual scans in a wide variety of tasks, with gradual increase in scan distance required. Here, improvements were reported on untrained tasks, including activities of daily living. A big change brought about by technology is that the *same* device (e.g. tablet) can change from being a book, to a movie viewer, to a camera, to a document one is writing, and so on. An exciting area for future research is whether there is spontaneous generalization of scanning gains from one trained tablet activity to another.

Limb activation

Attentional selection appears closely bound up in planning and executing action, and patients may show significantly less left neglect when using their left hands (Robertson and North, 1992; Samuel *et al.*, 2000). However, many patients who can make left limb movements fail to do so, they "neglect" their own actions. To counter this, Robertson *et al.* (1992) (see also Robertson *et al.*, 1998) developed a device to provide automatic movement reminders, such that periodic emitted tones were cancelled by left sided movement. Importantly, the benefits of limb activation training have been reported, in at least some cases, to extend beyond the cessation of training (e.g. O'Neill and McMillan, 2004). Mechanisms to account for this persistence include training movement habits or a positive feedback loop where increased awareness of the left (including the limb) increases spontaneous movements, which may account for the improvement in motor function up to 2-years post-training (Robertson *et al.*, 2002). Since these pioneering studies employing engineered devices, relevant technologies are more widespread. Smartphones, watches, and fitness-enhancing wristbands now contain very sensitive movement detectors (accelerometers) allowing the programming of new applications for these wearable consumer devices.

Hemifield patching and prism adaptation

A low-tech approach to retraining leftward eye movements was to ask patients to wear glasses that blanked off the *right* side of the world (Beis *et al.*, 1999). Participants were asked to wear the glasses for approximately 12 hours a day over three months (1,000 hours). Compared with a control group, there were significant increases in spontaneous leftward eye movements (when not wearing the glasses) and significant improvements in activities of daily living. A recent review (Smania *et al.*, 2013) notes variability in the reported outcomes, but concludes overall that there is evidence supporting clinical use. Monitoring of acceptability and user safety is recommended.

A conceptually similar approach is prism adaptation. Spectacles with thick Fresnel prismatic lenses distort light such that an object on the midline appears to be, for example, 10° to the right. When reaching to the apparent location, an initial 10° deviation of the hand is apparent. People quite rapidly adjust, such that when the glasses are removed, an error in the opposite direction often occurs for a short time. In a study in which patients with left neglect wore the glasses and made repeated points to various targets over five minutes, they showed this standard adaptation effect.

What was different and surprising, however, was that they also showed significantly improved awareness of the left for at least two hours post-training (Rossetti *et al.*, 1998). Replications followed, and in one study the effects of twice daily 20-minute prism adaptation (over two weeks) were still detectable six weeks later (Frassinetti *et al.*, 2002). Not all prism adaptation studies have demonstrated gains. A recent review concluded that more evidence was needed, particularly on maintenance and effects on functional performance of everyday tasks, before the relatively simple technology could be strongly recommended (Bowen *et al.*, 2013).

Neck muscle vibration

The brain integrates information from different sensory modalities in order to generate a working model of the world. Introducing a distortion to one stream (such as proprioception, the sense of relative location of one's limbs) can lead to bias in another (such as vision). The application of mechanical vibration to specific neck muscles can thus induce both a proprioceptive illusion of rotation and compensatory eye movements which reduce hemispatial neglect (Karnath *et al.*, 1993). In a randomized trial, Schindler *et al.* (2002) compared the effects of 15 40-minute sessions of spatial training with and without adjunct 80 Hz neck vibration. Practice alone had little detectable effect, whereas the addition of the vibration device produced gains on tests and measures of activities of daily living which were maintained at two months. Again, the application of a technology *obliging* patients to attend to left-space during spatial training increased their efficacy.

Transcranial magnetic stimulation (TMS) and transcranial direct current stimulation (tDCS)

In our awareness of space, the two hemispheres of the brain act in competition, the right hemisphere directing our attention to the left and the left hemisphere directing to the right. Thus, in unilateral lesions, we see both the effect of the lesion and the influence of the unaffected, unopposed hemisphere's dominance. Reports of spatial neglect being alleviated by a second stroke to the other hemisphere support this (e.g. Vuilleumier *et al.*, 1996) and have informed non-invasive brain stimulation/inhibition techniques in neglect rehabilitation. In TMS, an electric coil at the scalp produces a magnetic field, which, in turn, induces excitatory or inhibitory current in the underlying cortex. TMS induced inhibition of posterior regions of the right hemisphere can bring about left neglect-like phenomenon in healthy people, and TMS of the analogous intact left hemisphere regions can reduce manifestations of neglect (e.g. Muri *et al.*, 2013).

tDCS involves placement of large, plaster-like electrodes on the scalp between which a mild direct current is induced, modulating the excitability (how readily neurons will fire) of underlying cortex. Whilst at an early stage there are positive reports that tDCS, as TMS, can induce neglect-like phenomenon in healthy participants (Giglia *et al.*, 2011) and temporarily reduce neglect symptoms (Ko *et al.*,

2008), tDCS has advantages over TCS, requiring less specialized equipment, and being more acceptable and portable. Future scale clinical trials will answer how best to integrate tDCS with existing therapy and whether persisting effects generalize.

Alertness training

We have seen how the development and maintenance of a sufficiently alert state may be seen as a prerequisite for many attention and cognitive functions. When it comes to spatial attention, the relationship appears even more specific: patients with persistent left neglect tend to have problems in maintaining attention on many sorts of tasks (Robertson et al., 1997b; Samuelsson et al., 1998). Further, interventions designed to increase alertness, including loud tones, medication, and even placing time-pressure on task performance, have been shown to temporarily reduce left neglect (George et al., 2008; Malhotra et al., 2006; Robertson et al., 1998). In a repeated time-series design, Robertson and colleagues reported that self-alerting training (where participants develop a self-instructional strategy to be more alert) was linked with reductions in spatial bias, evident at least one day after training (Robertson et al., 1998). The support of self-instruction using wearable auditory prompting remains to be examined. Further work is required to develop and evaluate behavioral, biofeedback, pharmaceutical, and possibly non-invasive brain stimulation techniques to enhance alertness. This is potentially important, not just in neglect, but in enhancing the general attentional skills in a range of patient groups.

In summary, various technologies have been applied to the management of attention. These range from stimulation to increased alertness in states of altered consciousness, training of attention and alertness based on electroencephalography and electrodermal biofeedback, computerized cognitive training, and automated reminders to pay attention. In the spatial domain, technological adjuncts have included prompters to engage in leftward visual scans, cues to move the neglected limb, hemifield patches and prism lenses, muscle vibration, and various forms of non-invasive brain stimulation. The published evidence base inevitably lags some years behind the latest technological innovations and it is to potential developments that we now speculatively turn.

The future...

There is nothing quite like writing about future developments to make a chapter sound dated by the time it appears. However, there are some clear trends. Humans have long used things around them to "outsource" cognitive functions: calendars and watches help us keep track of the time, written notes and knots in handkerchiefs act as reminders, and, most of all, people and contexts help us to bring relevant thoughts and skills to mind. This trend has continued into the electronic age with smartphones and tablets. New apps that are designed to enhance organization and function appear almost daily. For example, reminders can be time activated or location activated, rather than trying to select the face of a friend from a crowd, we can let our phone find their phone and navigate us towards them. As devices are increasingly linked on the "internet of things" the consequences of poor attention may be increasingly offset (e.g. your phone tells you that you have neglected to turn the cooker off). Whilst some worry, often with little evidence, that engineered adjuncts to human cognition will reduce our capabilities, there are likely to be numerous advantages to people with reduced capacity because of brain injury or aging.

One clear trend is the migration of these technologies from the phone to "wearables." Smart watches relay information from the phone to the wrist for at-a-glance updates. Google Glass has the potential for some quite revolutionary changes. These glasses project information via a "heads up" display prism in the user's visual field, and present sound via bone conduction at the ear. Applications may include discrete context specific reminders as well as more general "pay attention" reminders. Perhaps the real potential from wearables will be the ability to monitor bodily variables (biometrics) and possibly (e.g. from pattern recognition of what worn cameras see) what the wearer is *doing*. In principle, for example, it may be possible to know both that the user is driving and, from eye-blinks, heart rate, and GSR, that they are drowsy, and then provide auditory and visual warnings (assuming that Google are not already driving the car!). Perhaps the most important part of these developments in interventions for attention is the ability to adapt and write software code that uses the extraordinary built-in capabilities of these devices rather than having to try to engineer from scratch.

The other big change offered by technology is the increasing potential for on-line cognitive assessment and tailored evidenced-based training, including cognitive training (such as WMT discussed earlier), but also educational, strategy development, and mood management approaches. Connections between training and the "internet of things" might mean that relevant messages from the training are delivered by context-aware wearables.

Of course, high technology is not everything. Wilson and Robertson (1992) describe a single case study in which a patient was concerned about inattention when reading following a brain injury. The patient was given a pile of matches and invited to move a match from one pile to the next each time he noticed that his attention had wandered from the text. Thus, the average time for which he could attend to reading was calculated. In the training phase, he was asked only to read for this short period with gradual increases if no lapse occurred, and decreases if attention lapsed. Over many weeks the patient achieved the target. The case usefully illustrates that we attend to complete particular meaningful *goals*. Where people complain of "poor attention" it is crucial to consider and focus on the goal that the poor attention compromises. Highly sophisticated technology may help to achieve that goal – or it could be something as simple as a box of matches.

References

Antonucci, G., Guariglia, C., Judica, A., Magnotti, L., Paolucci, S., Pizzamiglio, L., and Zoccolotti, P. (1995). Effectiveness of Neglect Rehabilitation in a Randomized Group Study. *Journal of Clinical and Experimental Neuropsychology*, 17: 383–89.

Arns, M., de Ridder, S., Strehl, U., Breteler, M., and Coenen, A. (2009). Efficacy of Neurofeedback Treatment in ADHD: The Effects on Inattention, Impulsivity and Hyperactivity: A Meta-Analysis. *Clinical EEG and Neurosciences*, 40(3): 180–89.

Baddeley, A. D. (1993). Working Memory or Working Attention. In A. D. Baddeley and L. Weiskrantz (eds), *Attention: Selection, Awareness and Control: A Tribute to Donald Broadbent* (pp. 152–70). Oxford, UK: Oxford University Press.

Beis, J. M., Andre, J. M., Baumgarten, A., and Challier, B. (1999). Eye Patching in Unilateral Spatial Neglect: Efficacy of Two Methods. *Archives of Physical Medicine and Rehabilitation*, 80: 71–6.

Bisiach, E. and Luzzatti, C. (1978). Unilateral Neglect of Representational Space. *Cortex*, 14: 129–33.

Bowen, A., Hazelton, C., Pollock, A., and Lincoln, N. B. (2013). Cognitive Rehabilitation for Spatial Neglect Following Stroke. *The Cochrane Database of Systematic Reviews*, 7: CD003586.

Buckner, R. L., Andrews-Hanna, J. R., and Schacter, D. L. (2008). The Brain's Default Network: Anatomy, Function and Relevance to Disease. *Annals of the New York Academy of Sciences*, 1124: 1–38.

Diller, L. and Weinberg, J. (1977). Hemi-inattention in Rehabilitation: The Evolution of a Rational Rehabilitation Program. In E. A. Weinstein and R. P. Friedland (eds), *Advances in Neurology* (Vol. 10). New York, NY: Raven Press.

Duffner, K. R., Mesulam, M. M., Scinto, L. F. M., Acar, D., Calvo, V., Faust, R., Chabrerie, A., Kennedy, B., and Holocomb, P. (2000). The Central Role of the Prefrontal Cortex in Directing Attention to Novel Events. *Brain*, 123: 923–39.

Duncan, J. (2006). EPS Mid-career Award 2004: Brain Mechanisms of Attention. *Quarterly Journal of Experimental Psychology*, 59: 2–27.

Fish, J., Evans, J. J., Nimmo, M., Martin, E., Kersel, D., Bateman, A., Wilson, B. A., and Manly, T. (2007). Rehabilitation of Executive Dysfunction Following Brain Injury: "Content-Free" Cueing Improves Everyday Prospective Memory Performance. *Neuropsychologia*, 45(6): 1318–30.

Frassinetti, F., Angeli, V., Meneghello, F., Avanzi, S., and Ladavas, E. (2002). Long-lasting Amelioration of Visuospatial Neglect by Prism Adaptation. *Brain*, 125: 608–23.

Gaston, E. T. (1968). Foreword. In E. T. Gaston (ed.), *Music in Therapy*. New York, NY: Macmillan.

George, M. S., Mercer, J. S., Walker, R., and Manly, T. (2008). A Demonstration of Endogenous Modulation of Unilateral Spatial Neglect: The Impact of Apparent Time-Pressure on Spatial Bias. *Journal of the International Neuropsychological Society*, 14(1): 33–41.

Giglia, G., Mattaliano, P., Puma, A., Rizzo, S., Fierro, B., and Brighina, F. (2011). Neglect-like Effects Induced by tDCS Modulation of Posterior Parietal Cortices in Healthy Subjects. *Brain Stimulation*, 4(4): 294–99.

Greco, E., Milewski-Lopez, A., van den Berg, F., McGuire, S., and Robertson, I. H. (2013). Evaluation of the Efficacy of a Self-Administered Biofeedback Aided Alertness Training Programme for Healthy Older Adults. *Abstracts of the 8th Annual Psychology, Health and Medicine Conference 4th April 2011, NUIG* (1107).

Holmes, J., Gathercole, S. E., and Dunning, D. L. (2009). Adaptive Training Leads to Sustained Enhancement of Poor Working Memory in Children. *Developmental Science*, 12(4): F9–15.

Husain, M. and Rorden, C. (2003). Non-Spatially Lateralized Mechanisms in Hemispatial Neglect. *Nature Reviews Neuroscience*, 4: 26–36.

James, W. (1890). *Principles of Psychology*. New York, NY: Holt.

Kallinen, K. and Ravaja, N. (2007). Comparing Speakers Versus Headphones in Listening to News from a Computer – Individual Differences And Psychophysiological Responses. *Computers in Human Behavior*, 23(1): 303–17.

Karnath, H. O., Christ, K., and Hartje, W. (1993). Decrease of Contralateral Neglect by Neck Muscle Vibration and Spatial Orientation of Trunk Midline. *Brain*, 116: 383–96.

Klingberg, T., Fernell, E., Olesen, P., Johnson, M., Gustafsson, P., Dahlström, K., Gillberg, C., Forssberg, H., and Westerberg, H. (2005). Computerized Training of Working Memory in Children with ADHD: A Randomized, Controlled Trial. *Journal of the American Academy of Child and Adolescent Psychiatry*, 44(2): 177–86.

Ko, M. H., Han, S. H., Park, S. H., Seo, J. H., and Kim, Y. H. (2008). Improvement of Visual Scanning After DC Brain Polarization of Parietal Cortex in Stroke Patients With Spatial Neglect. *Neuroscience Letters*, 448(2): 171–74.

Lawson, I. R. (1962). Visual-spatial Neglect in Lesions of the Right Cerebral Hemisphere. A Study in Recovery. *Neurology*, 12: 23–33.

Levine, B., Robertson, I. H., Clare, L., Carter, G., Hong, J., Wilson, B. A., Duncan, J., and Stuss, D. T. (2000). Rehabilitation of Executive Functioning: An Experimental-Clinical Validation of Goal Management Training. *Journal of the International Neuropsychological Society*, 6: 299–312.

Levine, B., Stuss, D. T., Winocur, G., Binns, M. A., Fahy, L., Mandic, M., Bridges, K., and Robertson, I. H. (2007). Cognitive Rehabilitation in the Elderly: Effects on Strategic Behavior in Relation to Goal Management. *Journal of the International Neuropsychological Society*, 13(1): 143–52.

Malhotra, P. A., Parton, A. D., Greenwood, R., and Husain, M. (2006). Noradrenergic Modulation of Space Exploration in Visual Neglect. *Annals of Neurology*, 59(1): 186–90.

Manly, T., Davison, B., Heutink, J., Galloway, M., and Robertson, I. H. (2000). Not Enough Time or Not Enough Attention?: Speed, Error and Self-maintained Control in the Sustained Attention to Response Test (SART). *Clinical Neuropsychological Assessment*, 3: 167–77.

Manly, T., Lewis, G. H., Robertson, I. H., Watson, P. C., and Datta, A. (2002). Coffee in the Cornflakes: Time-of-day as a Modulator of Executive Response Control. *Neuropsychologia*, 40(1): 1–6.

Manly, T., Heutink, J., Davison, B., Gaynord, B., Greenfield, E., Parr, A., Ridgeway, V., and Robertson, I. H. (2004). An Electronic Knot in the Handkerchief: "Content Free Cueing" and the Maintenance of Attentive Control. *Neuropsychological Rehabilitation*, 14(1/2): 89–116.

Miotto, E. C., Evans, J. J., de Lucia, M. C., and Scaff, M. (2009). Rehabilitation of Executive Dysfunction: A Controlled Trial of an Attention and Problem Solving Treatment Group. *Neuropsychological Rehabilitation*, 19(4): 517–40.

Monastra, V. J., Monastra, D. M., and George, S. (2002). The Effects of Stimulant Therapy, EEG Biofeedback, and Parenting Style on the Primary Symptoms of Attention-Deficit/ Hyperactivity Disorder. *Applied Psychophysiology & Biofeedback*, 27(4): 231–49.

Monastra, V. J., Lynn, S., Linden, M., Lubar, J. F., Gruzelier, J., and LaVaque, T. J. (2005). Electroencephalographic Biofeedback in the Treatment of Attention-Deficit/ Hyperactivity Disorder. *Applied Psychophysiology and Biofeedback*, 30(2): 95–114.

Morris, R., Griffiths, O., Le Pelley, M. E., and Weickert, T. (2012). Attention to Irrelevant Cues is Related to Positive Symptoms in Schizophrenia. *Schizophrenia Bulletin*, 38, doi:10.1093/schbul/sbr192.

Muri, R. M., Cazzoli, D., Nef, T., Mosimann, U. P., Hopfner, S., and Nyffeler, T. (2013). Non-Invasive Brain Stimulation in Neglect Rehabilitation: An Update. *Frontiers in Human Neuroscience*, 7: 248.

Novakovic-Agopian, T., Chen, A. J., Rome, S., Abrams, G., Castelli, H., Rossi, A. R., McKim, R., Hills, N., and D'Esposito, M. (2011). Rehabilitation of Executive Functioning with Training in Attention Regulation Applied to Individually Defined Goals: A Pilot Study Bridging Theory, Assessment and Treatment. *Journal of Head Trauma Rehabilitation*, 26(5): 325–38.

O'Connor, C., Robertson, I. H., and Levine, B. (2011). The Prosthetics of Vigilant Attention: Random Cuing Cuts Processing Demands. *Neuropsychology*, 25(4): 535–43.

O'Kelly, J., James, L., Palaniappan, R., Taborin, J., Fachner, J., and Magee, W. L. (2013). Neurophysiological and Behavioral Responses to Music Therapy in Vegetative and Minimally Conscious States. *Frontiers in Human Neuroscience*, 7: 884.

O'Neill, B. and McMillan, T. M. (2004). The Efficacy of Contralesional Limb Activation in Rehabilitation of Unilateral Hemiplegia and Visual Neglect: A Baseline-Intervention Study. *Neuropsychological Rehabilitation*, 14(4): 437–47.

Paolucci, S., Antonucci, G., Grasso, M. G., Bragoni, M., Coiro, P., De Angelis, D., Romana Fusco, F., Morelli, D., Venturiero, V., Troisi, E., and Pratesi, L. (2003). Functional Outcome of Ischemic and Hemorrhagic Stroke Patients After Inpatient Rehabilitation: A Matched Comparison. *Stroke*, 34(12): 2861–65.

Parasuraman, R. and Nestor, P. G. (1991). Attention and Driving Skills in Aging and Alzheimer's Disease. *Human Factors*, 33(5): 539–57.

Posner, M. L. and Petersen, S. E. (1990). The Attention System of the Human Brain. *Annual Review of Neuroscience*, 13: 25–42.

Poulton, E. C. (1977). Arousing Stresses Increase Vigilance. In R. R. Mackie (ed.), *Vigilance: Theory, Operational Performance and Physiological Correlates* (pp. 423–60). New York, NY: Plenum Press.

Rich, L. P. (2009). Prompting Self-monitoring with Assistive Technology to Increase Academic Engagement in Students with Attention-Deficit/Hyperactivity Disorder Symptoms. Unpublished PsyD thesis. New York, NY: Hofstra University.

Robertson, I. H. (1990). Does Computerized Cognitive Rehabilitation Work? A Review. *Aphasiology*, 4(4): 381–405.

Robertson, I. H. and North, N. (1992). Spatio-motor Cueing in Unilateral Neglect: The Role of Hemispace, Hand and Motor Activation. *Neuropsychologia*, 30: 553–63.

Robertson, I. H., North, N., and Geggie, C. (1992). Spatio-motor Cueing in Unilateral Neglect: Three Single Case Studies of its Therapeutic Effects. *Journal of Neurology, Neurosurgery and Psychiatry*, 55: 799–805.

Robertson, I. H., Manly, T., Andrade, J., Baddeley, B. T., and Yiend, J. (1997a). Oops! Performance Correlates of Everyday Attentional Failures in Traumatic Brain Injured and Normal Subjects. *Neuropsychologia*, 35: 747–58.

Robertson, I. H., Manly, T., Beschin, N., Daini, R., Haeske-Deswick, H., Homberg, V., Jehkonen, M., Pizzamiglio, G., Shiel, A., and Weber, E. (1997b), Auditory Sustained Attention is a Marker of Unilateral Spatial Neglect. *Neuropsychologia*, 35(12): 527–532.

Robertson, I. H., Mattingley, J. B., Rorden, C., and Driver, J. (1998). Phasic Alerting of Neglect Patients Overcomes Their Spatial Deficit in Visual Awareness. *Nature*, 395: 169–72.

Robertson, I. H., McMillan, T. M., MacLeod, E., Edgeworth, J., and Brock, D. (2002). Rehabilitation by Limb Activation Training (LAT) Reduces Impairment in Unilateral Neglect Patients: A Single Blind Randomised Control Trial. *Neuropsychological Rehabilitation*, 12: 439–54.

Rossetti, Y., Rode, G., Pisella, L., Farne, A., Li, L., Boisson, D., and Perenin, M. T. (1998). Prism Adaptation to a Rightward Optical Deviation Rehabilitates Left Hemispatial Neglect. *Nature*, 395: 166–69.

Samuel, C., Louis-Dreyfus, A., Kaschel, R., Makiela, E., Troubat, M., Anselmi, N., Cannizzo, V., and Azouvi, P. (2000). Rehabilitation of Very Severe Unilateral Neglect by Visuo-Spatio-Motor Cueing: Two Single Case Studies. *Neuropsychological Rehabilitation*, 10(4): 385–99.

Samuelsson, H., Hjelmquist, E., Jensen, C., Ekholm, S., and Blomstrand, C. (1998). Non-lateralized Attentional Deficits: An Important Component Behind Persisting Visuospatial Neglect? *Journal of Clinical and Experimental Neuropsychology*, 20(1): 73–88.

Schindler, I., Kerkhoff, G., Karnath, H.-O., Keller, I., and Goldenberg, G. (2002). Neck Muscle Vibration Induces Lasting Recovery in Spatial Neglect. *Journal of Neurology, Neurosurgery and Psychiatry*, 73: 412–19.

Smania, N., Fonte, C., Picelli, A., Gandolfi, M., and Varalta, V. (2013). Effect of Eye Patching in Rehabilitation of Hemispatial Neglect. *Frontiers in Human Neuroscience*, 7(527). Available at: www.ncbi.nlm.nih.gov/pmc/articles/PMC3759299/ (accessed 28 July 2014).

Sörqvist, P. (2010). The Role of Working Memory Capacity in Auditory Distraction: A Review. *Theoretical Aspects of Auditory Distraction*, 12(49): 217–24.

Spira, E. G. and Fischel, J. E. (2005). The Impact of Preschool Inattention, Hyperactivity, and Impulsivity on Social and Academic Development: A Review. *Journal of Child Psychology and Psychiatry*, 46(7): 755–73.

Steriade, M. (1996). Arousal: Revisiting the Reticular Activating System. *Science*, 272(5259): 225–26.

Sterzi, R., Bottini, G., Celani, M. G., Righetti, E., Lamassa, M., Ricci, S., and Vallar, G. (1993). Hemianopia, Hemianaesthesia and Hemiplegia after Right and Left Hemispheric Damage. A Hemispheric Difference. *Journal of Neurology, Neurosurgery and Psychiatry*, 56: 308–10.

Stone, S. P., Patel, P., and Greenwood, R. J. (1993). Selection of Acute Stroke Patients for Treatment of Visual Neglect. *Journal of Neurology, Neurosurgery, and Psychiatry*, 56(5): 463–66.

Thatcher, R. W. (2000). EEG Operant Conditioning (Biofeedback) and Traumatic Brain Injury. *Clinical Electroencephalography*, 31(1): 38–44.

Underbjerg, M., George, M. S., Thorsen, P., Kesmodel, U. S., Mortensen, E. L., and Manly, T. (2013). Separable Sustained and Selective Attention Factors Are Apparent in 5-year-old Children. *PLoS one*, 8(12): e82843.

Vuilleumier, P., Hester, D., Assal, G., and Regli, F. (1996). Unilateral Spatial Neglect Recovery After Sequential Strokes. *Neurology*, 19: 184–89.

Westerberg, H., Jacobaeus, H., Hirvikoski, T., Clevberger, P., Ostensson, M., Bartfai, A., and Klingberg, T. (2007). Computerized Working Memory Training After Stroke: A Pilot Study. *Brain Injury*, 21(1): 21–9.

Wilson, C. and Robertson, I. H. (1992). A Home-Based Intervention for Attentional Slips During Reading Following Head Injury: A Single Case Study. *Neuropsychological Rehabilitation*, 2: 193–205.

Wilson, S. L., Cranny, S., and Andrews, K. (1992). The Efficacy of Music for Stimulation in Prolonged Coma: Four Single Case Experiments. *Clinical Rehabilitation*, 6: 181–87.

Yerkes, R. M. and Dodson, J. D. (1908). The Relation of Strength of Stimulus to Rapidity of Habit-Formation. *Journal of Comparative Neurology and Psychology*, 18: 459–82.

3

ASSISTIVE TECHNOLOGY FOR MEMORY

Bonnie-Kate Dewar, Michael Kopelman,
Narinder Kapur, and Barbara A. Wilson

Memory impairment commonly occurs after acquired brain injury, such as traumatic brain injury, stroke, or encephalitis, and can have a negative impact upon an individual's ability to live independently and return to his or her premorbid level of community participation (Ben-Yishay and Diller, 1993; Sohlberg, 2005) as well as having a potentially devastating effect on adjustment to the brain injury with subsequent mood and anxiety disorders (Tate, 2002).

Memory has been understood in terms of semantic, episodic, and working memory systems (see Bradley *et al.*, 2005). Episodic memory refers to the encoding, storage, and utilization of personally experienced events that can be related to specific temporal and spatial contexts. Semantic memory refers to an organized body of knowledge about words, concepts, and culturally and educationally acquired facts. Working memory refers to the ability to hold and manipulate information in a temporary store over a period of seconds. Other memory systems are largely independent of conscious recollection and include the implicit memory processes of procedural memory. This is the ability to acquire new skills or utilize previously acquired skills. It is also important to note that the process of remembering can be broken down into the stages of encoding, storage and consolidation, and retrieval (Bradley *et al.*, 2005). One form of recall that is particularly relevant to the everyday impact of memory impairments is that of prospective memory, which is the ability to remember an intended action at some time in the future.

Rehabilitation techniques have been developed to manage memory difficulties. The ultimate goal of rehabilitation is to enable people to function as independently as possible in their own most appropriate environment (McLellan, 1991). One of the ways this can be achieved is through the use of compensatory memory aids. A range of memory aids are now available, can be inexpensive, and have the potential to be highly effective in the compensation of memory problems. Rehabilitation can enable people with brain injury to bypass or reduce cognitive deficits in order to function as adequately as possible in an environment that is most appropriate to them (Wilson and Evans, 2003). This reflects the World Health Organization's International Classification of Functioning, Disability and Health (2001) which focuses upon the impact of an impairment on an individual's ability to function and limitations on participation. With respect to memory rehabilitation, such a framework suggests that we need to identify any strategy or technique that will assist individuals with acquired memory disorders to actively function and participate in their desired environment.

Compensatory approaches to memory impairment seek to bypass the deficit area and teach the individual how to use certain strategies to solve functional problems (Kapur and Wilson 2009). With mastery of compensatory strategies, this approach assumes that the individual will be able to manage in their everyday environment despite the presence of the underlying impairment. External memory aids are the most effective and widely used intervention for the rehabilitation of memory impairments (Sohlberg, 2005; Sohlberg et al., 2007b). An external memory aid is a tool or device that "either limits the demands on the person's impaired ability or transforms the task or environment such that it matches the client's abilities" (Sohlberg, 2005: 51). Use of at least six compensatory memory aids has been associated with increased independence, as defined by being in paid employment, full time education, living alone, or taking a major role in running the household/caring for children (Wilson and Watson, 1996; Evans et al., 2003). A large variety of memory aids have been described in the literature, with varying degrees of technical complexity. There are many paper-and-pencil or low technology aids, including notebooks, diaries, and calendars, which are commonly used (Evans et al., 2003).

Although this chapter concentrates on the more "high-tech" electronic aids, we will say a few words about the stationery-based aids. Memory notebooks and diaries successfully compensate for a variety of functional tasks, including circumventing impairments in prospective memory (Sohlberg and Mateer, 1989; Fleming et al., 2005; Shum et al., 2011) – the ability to remember to carry out an action at a specific time in the future. A distinction has been made between event-based prospective tasks (post the letter when you see a post box), time-based tasks (take your medication at 10 a.m.) or activity-based tasks (take your medication after brushing your teeth). It has been suggested that compensatory aids, such as stationery-based items, support prospective memory by both transforming event-based tasks into time-based prospective tasks (Jeong and Cranney, 2009) and then triggering the intention that something has to be done and retrieving the content of what has to be done (Fleming et al., 2005). Memory aids can also support general prospective goals, such as completing a task at some time in the future, in addition to specific tasks that need to be completed at a set time (Fish et al., 2010).

High-technology memory aids

Whilst low-technology stationery memory aids have been widely available for many decades, there is a rapidly growing market of high-technology electronic memory aids. Examples include timers, calendars operated on a personal computer, personal data assistants (PDAs), smartphones, voice recorders, watches with alarms, and paging devices (see Hermann *et al.*, 1999; Kapur *et al.*, 2004; Kapur and Wilson, 2009). Given that many everyday memory difficulties, in both brain injured and non-neurological populations, are prospective memory difficulties with problems remembering to carry out future intentions (Fish *et al.*, 2010), electronic memory aids have the potential to remind the user not only what they have to do, but also when they have to do it. A survey of over 1,000 patients suffering from multiple sclerosis found that around half of them used electronic memory aids (Johnson *et al.*, 2009). Some memory-impaired people are unwilling to use such aids, however, and, as Baldwin *et al.* (2011) note, "The motivation to use strategies depends on more complex processes that include social, emotional, and practical factors, all of which need to be considered and are potentially modifiable" (2011: 499). Another problem is that there can be difficulty in both learning and remembering to use electronic reminders. Nevertheless, even densely amnesic patients can sometimes use electronic devices to help them function in everyday life (Wilson, 2009).

NeuroPage

One of the most compelling sets of evidence for the rehabilitation of (prospective) memory function with the use of compensatory memory aids comes from a series of studies using an alpha-numeric paging system to target specific everyday functional goals. The NeuroPage system (Wilson *et al.*, 1997; Wilson *et al.*, 2003) has been shown to assist people with memory and planning problems following acquired brain injury to carry out everyday tasks. After selection of target behaviors, such as remembering to take medication or attendance at appointments, participants were provided with a pager and then sent reminders for these behaviors at times agreed with the participant and their caregiver. With a sample of 143 participants, use of the pager significantly increased performance of target behaviors relative to baseline (Wilson *et al.*, 1997; Wilson *et al.*, 2001).

The use of the pager has been examined with respect to a participant's aetiology, with successful use in participants with traumatic brain injury (Wilson *et al.*, 2005), encephalitis (Emslie *et al.*, 2007), and cerebrovascular disease (Fish *et al.*, 2008b). NeuroPage has also been successfully used in a group of children and adolescents (Wilson *et al.*, 2009). A recent review of the NeuroPage service considered use of the device alongside growing accessibility to mobile and smartphone technology (Martin-Saez *et al.*, 2011). The authors concluded that the paging service continued to have a role within cognitive rehabilitation as either a long-term cognitive prosthetic for people with more severe cognitive and behavioral problems or as a tool to assist people to use technology to foster independence early in their rehabilitation. NeuroPage has been specifically used to compensate for the impact of executive dysfunction on everyday behaviors in a woman recovering from stroke (Evans *et al.*, 1998). A review of this case study (Fish *et al.*, 2008a) confirmed the utility of specific goal-related messages in addition to a more general prompt to review activities. NeuroPage is purported to support memory by provision of information about what a client has to do in addition to provision of an alert which acts to focus attention and assist goal review (Fish *et al.*, 2008a). Indeed, an individual with both memory and executive dysfunction may benefit from additional executive strategy training in combination with use of the paging system (Fish *et al.*, 2008a).

Voice recorders

Another form of electronic memory aid is a portable Dictaphone-type device that can replay messages at a time and date specified by the user. Van den Broek *et al.* (2000) used a Voice Organiser recorder, which alerted the user to play a previously recorded message with an auditory alert at a specified time and date. Prospective memory for everyday tasks, including passing a message to a caregiver, was improved for a group of five people with brain injury. A similar recording device, a Sony IC Recorder, was used to record therapy tasks, such as completing a diary, in a group of patients following stroke or traumatic brain injury (TBI) (Yasuda *et al.*, 2002). Experimenter-recorded messages were heralded at a set time by an alarm followed by the message, and resulted in increased completion of targeted daily tasks. Use of a Voice Craft voice recorder in combination with written reminders was instigated to address medication compliance in an individual with significant memory and executive impairments following TBI (Van Hulle and Hux, 2006). Use of the voice recorder was not successful, possibly because of poor motivation to increase independence. This patient also did not benefit from the use of a Watchminder, a wrist-watch alarm with written prompt, in contrast to another subject who was able to use this memory aid to independently manage his medication regime. Additionally, Oriani *et al.* (2003) successfully used a voice recorder to improve completion of everyday prospective memory tasks in a group of people with mild to moderate dementia. The voice recorder was shown to be superior to written reminders, and patients were provided with specific training in the use of the memory aid. Voice prompts have also been effective in increasing medication adherence in a sample of subjects with HIV infection and memory impairment (Andrade *et al.*, 2001). The Disease Management Assistance System was programmed to sound an alert and play a message when a dose of medication was due, and a record was kept of the time and date when the medication was taken.

Electronic organizers

Portable electronic organizers were an early form of technology used to support memory function. Giles and Shore (1989) demonstrated the superiority of a Psion organizer to a paper-based organizer to facilitate completion of everyday tasks for a woman recovering from a subarachnoid hemorrhage. The organizer had an electronic diary function with an alarm in addition to a "memo pad" command for storing miscellaneous information. PDAs containing a diary, notebook, and a to-do-list were found to be useful by a group of people with acquired brain injury

(Wright *et al.*, 2001). PDA use was also found to be superior to written lists or a paper-based planner in a group of students with traumatic brain injury (Gillette and DePompei, 2004). Interestingly, the students were not required to enter details of the experimental prospective memory tasks, only to familiarize themselves with the device. Gentry *et al.* (2008) investigated the use of an off-the-shelf Palm PDA as a cognitive aid in a group of people with traumatic brain injury. Training was provided in how to use the calendar, alarm, appointments, and tasks ("to do") functions on the PDA. Following two months of use, participants reported improved performance and satisfaction with performance in everyday tasks in addition to increased levels of participation in areas of cognition, mobility, and occupation (Gentry *et al.*, 2008). More recently, Dowds *et al.* (2011) compared the effectiveness of a paper-based memory aid to PDA/Palm top memory aids in 36 subjects with traumatic brain injury. Participants were given an experimental prospective memory task and three personal tasks to complete using the low- or high-technology memory aids. Although the exact training was not specified, use of an electronic memory aid with an alarm increased the rate of timely task completion in survivors of TBI with self-reported memory problems. Similar benefits for prospective memory using a Palm top PDA have been reported (Waldron *et al.*, 2012). A randomized control trial that compared a PDA with paper-and-pencil diary training found that both were of benefit in areas such as goal attainment, but they did not find a significant difference between the two interventions (De Joode *et al.*, 2013) – factors such as patient selection and treatment procedure differences may help to explain the differences between the Dowds *et al.* and the De Joode *et al.* studies.

Mobile phones and smartphone technology

Mobile phones are increasingly attractive as "high-tech" memory aids as their use becomes ubiquitous in the non-neurologically injured population. Mobile phones also have the advantage of being portable, potentially cost effective, and more socially acceptable. The reminder functions in such phones have been found to improve compliance in a number of healthcare settings (Prasad and Anand, 2012; Hasvold and Wootton, 2011; Horvath *et al.*, 2012).

Mobile phones were initially used as reminding devices in rehabilitation, with evaluation of the use of SMS text messages to prompt execution of prospective tasks. An early study into the use of a "standard" mobile phone incorporated a reminder message sent to the participant's phone to act as a memory prompt for completion of everyday tasks. Compared to self-initiated performance, reminders sent to a mobile phone increased initiation of everyday tasks such as taking medication or self-care tasks (Wade and Troy, 2001), addressing difficulties in memory, planning, and organization. Stapleton *et al.* (2007) provided mobile phones programmed with individualized messages using a reminder function. Written reminder messages appeared on the phone in conjunction with an auditory tone at a specified time and date. However, use of these mobile phone reminders was not successful in increasing performance of target behaviors in subjects with severe memory impairments (Stapleton *et al.*, 2007). SMS text messages facilitated recall of rehabilitation therapy goals (Culley and Evans, 2010), with a general alerting effect that generalized to other non-targeted therapy goals. Similarly, participants with organizational problems following acquired brain injury were sent randomly timed text messages to prompt goal review and improve prospective memory function (Fish *et al.*, 2007). The messages were a mnemonic form of brief goal management training and served to enhance general prospective memory function. Pijnenborg *et al.* (2007) demonstrated that short text messages increase achievement of personally selected everyday goals in a sample of people with schizophrenia. The treatment effect was dependent on continuous use of the mobile phone and more pronounced in subjects with more severe impairments at baseline.

The advent of "smartphone" technology has provided an electronic memory aid that encompasses PDA capabilities within a mobile phone. Smartphones, utilizing built-in reminders, were more effective in facilitating task completion, compared with a paper-based planner, for adolescents and adults with traumatic brain injury (DePompei *et al.*, 2008). The authors suggested that the audible reminder may have accounted for the success of the smartphone not only for specific tasks but also to prompt use of the memory aid itself – "use your reminder." The most common functions used by subjects were organizational and communication tools, such as the calendar, contacts, and task lists, in addition to the camera and games.

The relentless advance of smartphone technology has presented a challenge to provide evidence of the effectiveness of smartphones in memory rehabilitation research. Svoboda *et al.* (2012) have developed a theoretical-based training program to support people with moderate to severe memory problems to use smartphones and PDAs. Based upon Sohlberg and Mateer's (1989) model of memory compensation training, the authors suggest that the training approach can be applied to any number of emerging technologies. Training comprised two phases: acquisition of skills to use the calendar function of the smartphone or PDA, and then real life generalization. The calendar application was broken down into component steps and trained with the error reduction technique of vanishing cues. Once a criterion of successful use of the calendar application was achieved, subjects practiced entering events into the calendar, making plans, and attaching notes. Generalization occurred within the home to apply the skills to a real life setting. Training continued until skill acquisition and generalization were successful rather than after a set number of sessions (Svoboda *et al.*, 2012). Ten subjects with acquired memory disorders demonstrated improved day-to-day memory function following training. These subjects included two cases that had been previously described – one subject with amnesia following removal of a colloid cyst (Svoboda and Richards, 2009) and a young adult with a severe memory impairment following treatment of a suprasellar germinoma at the age of 13 (Svoboda *et al.*, 2010). The effective use of smartphone technology was maintained over an 18-month period for the subject with amnesia following the removal of a colloid cyst (Savage and Svoboda, 2013).

Recent developments in mobile phone technology include platforms for the optimal use of Windows applications, email, web browsing, GPS maps and adoption of so-called "third generation" applications (or apps). Whilst apps are available for "brain training" and memory training drills, as noted above there is little evidence to support the use of repetitive drills in the rehabilitation of everyday memory problems (see Wilson, 2009). Rather, it is the (rapid) development of apps that act as a support to everyday memory function that may hold the most promise for use with people with memory and other cognitive impairments following acquired brain injury. These include apps that act as reminders on the basis of both time and location, supports to locate personal belongings, medication adherence, academic study supports, or organizational programs which provide voice prompts to initiate everyday tasks. However, the proliferation of apps stands in contrast to compensatory devices carefully developed and tested. Clinicians need to determine the efficacy of available apps. The additional challenge for the clinician is the development of a methodology for training in the use of the smartphone and associated apps in addition to keeping up to date with these rapid technological developments. In this respect, Svoboda and colleagues' training program (2009, 2010) described above is an exciting development, particularly given its success with subjects with severe memory impairments. Similarly, a manual has been produced for use of an iPod Touch, iPhone, and iPad as a memory/cognitive prosthetic device following acquired brain injury (Wild, 2011; see www.id4theweb.com). The program, based upon a training program for a Windows-based mobile device (Wild and Schwartz, 2009), systematically trains specific skills to use these smart devices, whilst attempting to generalize these skills to other real-world tasks.

Software to guide performance

O'Neill *et al.* (2010) distinguish between scheduling support, which provides reminders regarding when to perform tasks, and sequencing support, where expert systems guide performance in everyday tasks. The use of smartphones as a compensatory memory aid is an example of a scheduling-assistive technology device. A number of software packages have been developed to minimize the cognitive challenges presented in specific everyday tasks and provide interactive "scaffolding" to compensate for memory or executive impairments (Cole, 1999; LoPresti *et al.*, 2004). These include the Planning and Execution Assistant and Training System (PEAT, see Levinson, 1997), which generates the best plan to complete steps required in a task with the support of visual and auditory cues, and COACH (Cognitive Orthosis for Assisting activities at Home; Boger and Mihailidis, 2011) which has been used to support people with dementia to complete hand washing independently. More recently, commercial products, such as Pocket Coach provided by AbleLink (Gentry *et al.*, 2008), create a step-by-step sequence of visual cues on a desktop computer that are then loaded onto a PDA to aid task completion. Similarly, use of ICue (LoPresti *et al.*, 2008), an interactive software program presented on a PDA, reduced the number of errors in everyday tasks in two subjects with acquired brain injury by the provision of visual/graphic cues in addition to written text. Future developments of these cognitive support systems include the ability to recognize different situations and adapt to the individual's needs. For example, a context-aware medication reminding program that waits until the individual is not otherwise engaged to prompt medication use (Boger and Mihailidis, 2011).

Other technologies

To overcome the cost associated with the use of technological memory aids, McDonald et al. (2011) conducted a randomized controlled trial of Google Calendar, an electronic calendar available free of charge on the Internet, with the advantage that timed text reminders can be sent directly to a client's mobile phone. The calendar is easy to use as it only requires events to be entered into the calendar, noting the date and time the reminder is required and selecting the reminder message. Subjects with an acquired brain injury were required to use weekly record charts to monitor completion of prospective memory tasks. Compared to standard diary use, Google Calendar was shown to be significantly more effective than a paper-based diary in supporting subjects' prospective intentions (McDonald et al., 2011). The results were interpreted as positive support for the use of this technology for people with acquired memory and executive disorders and in support of active reminders over passive reminders, such as paper-based diaries, calendars, or notes.

Technology allows for novel approaches to support independent living and compensate for memory problems within an individual's environment. Lemoncello and Prideaux (2011) conducted a randomized controlled trial of Television Assisted Prompting (TAP). This system consisted of a set-top box positioned close to the client's home television with which they interact using their remote control. The TAP system turns on the television at any time to deliver reminders that have been programmed remotely from a computer. Compared to brain injured clients' typical memory prompts, the TAP system allowed completion of a greater number of tasks and improved confidence (Lemoncello and Prideaux, 2011). Task completion improved from 43 percent during the typical reminder period to 72 percent task completion with the support of the TAP system.

One platform which brings together a number of emerging technologies is the "Smart Home," a living environment constructed to assist people with disabilities carry out everyday activities by using various integrated assistive technology systems (Dewsbury and Linskell, 2011), such as turning off electrical equipment or sensors to monitor wandering. Boman et al. (2007) trained eight people, with memory impairments secondary to traumatic brain injury or stroke, in the use of a number of electronic aids. These included electronic keys, a stove guard, a remote control which activates lights and power to kitchen equipment, and a lap top with email alerts and an electronic calendar. Training was conducted in situ and consisted of breaking each task into a sequence of steps, then training each step with errorless learning principles. In a similar "smart house" apartment, Boman et al. (2010) instructed 14 subjects, with moderate memory impairments following traumatic brain injury or stroke, to use a number of electronic memory aids. Memory aids included a daily computer-based schedule, equipment control panels, and kitchen alarms. Dewsbury and Linskell (2011) have suggested a neurological dependability assessment matrix to facilitate the technological-fit of smart house technology to the needs and wishes of the individual with the neurological condition.

An emerging compensatory aid for support of autobiographical memory is the use of a wearable camera, which passively records images throughout the day, automatically or during selected events (Hodges *et al.*, 2011). The images are then reviewed as a pictorial diary at a later time, akin to watching a movie of the event or day. Developed by Microsoft under the brand name SenseCam, this technology was made commercially available as Vicon Revue (www.viconrevue.com), and has now been replaced by a similar device (www.autographer.com). In an initial case study of a woman recovering from limbic encephalitis, recall of autobiographical events with SenseCam with a delay of one day was superior to the use of a written diary (Berry *et al.*, 2007). Recall was maintained across a delay of 11 months. It is suggested that, with this case, SenseCam images functioned to facilitate consolidation of episodes into long-term memory by promoting activation of frontal and posterior cortical regions (Berry *et al.*, 2009). Alternatively, SenseCam may facilitate recall of otherwise inaccessible episodic memories through the capture of images from the perspective of the individual and the temporal ordering of images (Loveday and Conway, 2011). With the presentation of a large number of images, and thus a wide range of related but changing visual cues, SenseCam also increases the likelihood that the record of the event contains an effective cue.

SenseCam has shown promise in a cognitive behavioral therapeutic intervention in a young man experiencing social anxiety subsequent to a TBI (Brindley *et al.*, 2011). The device appeared to support retrieval of personally salient anxiety-provoking events with reference to internal states. SenseCam also increased the long-term retention of specific episodes in a 13-year-old boy with anterograde amnesia secondary to a brain tumor treated with radio and chemotherapy (Pauly-Takacs *et al.*, 2011). It was suggested that review of the SenseCam images facilitated the formation of personal semantic memories. Future developments in the use of wearable memory prostheses include context-aware memory devices (LoPresti *et al.*, 2004) to extend location-based reminders to include information such as person identification and additional semantic information about social environments (see Vemuri and Bender, 2004; Kikhia *et al.*, 2009).

Other emerging technologies include the use of touch screens and touch tablets to promote reminiscence therapy in people with dementia (Astell *et al.*, 2010; Lloyd-Yeates, 2013), and the use of virtual reality to help Alzheimer's Disease patients relearn everyday skills such as cooking (Yamaguchi *et al.*, 2012).

Clinical case

Bateman (unpublished) described a 50-year-old woman who had sustained anoxic brain damage following a myocardial infarction three years earlier. She was left with significant prospective memory problems, restricting her level of independence.

However, as she regularly used her mobile phone, it was decided to send text messages in an attempt to help her achieve everyday tasks. In addition to written messages, mobile phones can be used to send pictures, photographs, and even videos, so they have greater potential than other systems, such as pagers. Nine main problems were identified to do with medication, security, and cooking. During the first week, daily baselines were taken on the achievement of these behaviors; in weeks two to four, reminder texts were sent at agreed times and on agreed days. In week five, the text messages were randomly and partially withdrawn. In week six, no messages were sent.

Total achievement of all behaviors was 59 percent during the baseline, increasing to 97 percent during week four. This was maintained (98 percent) when the messages were partially withdrawn and showed a slight decrease to 93 percent when the messages stopped. These results can be seen in Figures 3.1, 3.2, and 3.3.

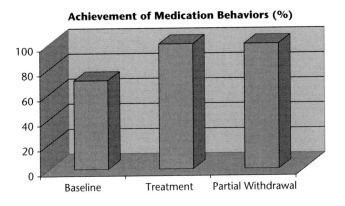

FIGURE 3.1 Medication behaviors

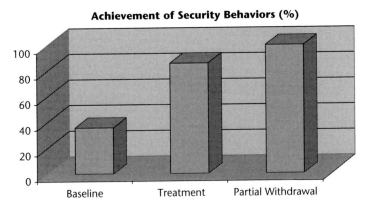

FIGURE 3.2 Security behaviors (e.g. remembering to lock doors)

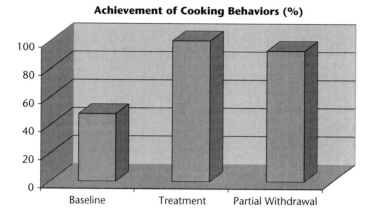

Achievement of Cooking Behaviors (%)

FIGURE 3.3 Cooking behaviors

Conclusions

There is a growing body of evidence that supports the effectiveness of external compensatory memory aids to improve the everyday function of people with memory impairments (Sohlberg *et al.*, 2007a). Gillespie *et al.* (2012) suggest a novel but practical conceptualization for assistive technologies for cognition (ATC) in terms of functionality within which the application of memory aids in cognitive rehabilitation can be understood. The authors classify the functions of ATC devices in terms of ICF cognitive functions (World Health Organization, 2001) with a literature review which suggests that time management is supported by prompting devices, episodic memory by devices which store and display large amounts of information, and organization and planning by interactive prompting devices. This approach moves away from the use of specific devices to a consideration of the generalizable level of ATC function in cognitive terms, and facilitates the measurement of treatment outcome in terms of changes in activity and participation. For example, the authors cite the strong evidence of the NeuroPage study (Wilson *et al.*, 2001) as evidence for a reminding ATC. This framework thus helps clinicians to select and appropriately match memory aids to their client's needs, whilst considering the impact upon activity and, ultimately, participation. Future areas for memory aid development include technology to support person recognition; to include storage and flexible retrieval of face, name, and semantic information. In addition, whilst Autographer shows promise, a future challenge for such technology is the development of software that will enable video and other photographic records to be easily archived and retrieved, and thus allow an interface between sophisticated data retrieval systems and online records. A remaining challenge is the development of an effective approach to the systematic training in the use of memory aids in rehabilitation.

References

Andrade, A. S., McGruder, H. F., Wu, A. W., Celano, S. A., Skolasky Jr, R. L., Selnes, O. A., Huang, I. C., and McArthur, J. C. (2001). A Programmable Prompting Device Improves Adherence to Highly Active Antiretroviral Therapy in HIV-Infected Subjects with Memory Impairment. *Clinical Infectious Diseases*, 41(6): 875–82.

Astell, A., Ellis, M., Bernardi, L., Alm, N., Dye, R., Gowans, G., and Campbell, J. (2010). Using a Touch Screen Computer to Support Relationships Between People with Dementia and Caregivers. *Interacting with Computers*, 22(4): 267–75.

Baldwin, V., Powell, T., and Lorenc, L. (2011). Factors Influencing the Uptake of Memory Compensations: A Qualitative Analysis. *Neuropsychological Rehabilitation*, 21: 484–501.

Ben-Yishay, Y. and Diller, L. (1993). Cognitive Remediation in Traumatic Brain Injury: Update and Issues. *Archives of Physical Medicine and Rehabilitation*, 74(2): 204–13.

Berry, E., Kapur, N., Williams, L., Hodges, S., Watson, P., Smyth, G., Srinivasan, J., Smith, R., Wilson, B., and Wood, K. (2007). The Use of a Wearable Camera, SenseCam, as a Pictorial Diary to Improve Autobiographical Memory in a Patient with Limbic Encephalitis: A Preliminary Report. *Neuropsychological Rehabilitation*, 17(4–5): 582–601.

Berry, E., Hampshire, A., Rowe, J., Hodges, S., Kapur, N., Watson, P., Browne, G., Smyth, G., Wood, K., and Owen, A. (2009). The Neural Basis of Effective Memory Therapy in a Patient with Limbic Encephalitis. *Journal of Neurology, Neurosurgery and Psychiatry*, 80(11): 1202–05.

Boger, J. and Mihailidis, A. (2011). The Future of Intelligent Assistive Technologies for Cognition: Devices Under Development to Support Independent Living and Aging-With-Choice. *NeuroRehabilitation*, 28(3): 271–80.

Boman, I.-L., Tham, K., Granqvist, A., Bartfai, A., and Hemmingsson, H. (2007). Using Electronic Aids to Daily Living After Acquired Brain Injury: A Study of the Learning Process and the Usability. *Disability and Rehabilitation. Assistive Technology*, 2(1): 23–33.

Boman, I.-L., Lindberg Stenvall, C., Hemmingsson, H., and Bartfai, A. (2010). A Training Apartment with a Set of Electronic Memory Aids for Patients with Cognitive Problems. *Scandinavian Journal of Occupational Therapy*, 17(2): 140–48.

Bradley, V., Kapur, N., and Evans, J. J. (2005). Memory Assessment in Memory Rehabilitation. In Halligan, P. and Wade, D. T. (eds), *Rehabilitation of Cognitive Deficits* (pp. 115–34). Oxford, UK: Oxford University Press.

Brindley, R., Bateman, A., and Gracey, F. (2011). Exploration of Use of SenseCam to Support Autobiographical Memory Retrieval within a Cognitive-Behavioural Therapeutic Intervention Following Acquired Brain Injury. *Memory*, 19(7): 745–57.

Cole, E. (1999). Cognitive Prosthetics: An Overview to a Method of Treatment. *NeuroRehabilitation*, 12: 39–51.

Culley, C. and Evans, J. J. (2010). SMS Text Messaging as a Means of Increasing Recall of Therapy Goals in Brain Injury Rehabilitation: A Single-Blind Within-Subjects Trial. *Neuropsychological Rehabilitation*, 20(1): 103–19.

De Joode, E., Van Heugten, C., Verhey, F., and Van Boxtel, M. (2013). Effectiveness of an Electronic Cognitive Aid in Patients with Acquired Brain Injury: A Multi-Centre Randomised Parallel-Group Study. *Neuropsychological Rehabilitation*, 23: 133–56.

DePompei, R., Gillette, Y., Goetz, E., Xenopoulos-Oddsson, A., Bryen, D., and Dowds, M. (2008). Practical Applications for Use of PDAs and Smartphones with Children and Adolescents Who Have Traumatic Brain Injury. *NeuroRehabilitation*, 23(6): 487–99.

Dewsbury, G. and Linskell, J. (2011). Smart Home Technology for Safety and Functional Independence: The UK Experience. *NeuroRehabilitation*, 28(3): 249–60.

Dowds, M. M., Lee, P. H., Sheer, J. B., O'Neil-Pirozzi, T. M., Xenopoulos-Oddsson, A., Goldstein, R., Zainea, K. L., and Glenn, M. B. (2011). Electronic Reminding Technology Following Traumatic Brain Injury: Effects on Timely Task Completion. *The Journal of Head Trauma Rehabilitation*, 26(5): 339–47.

Emslie, H., Wilson, B. A., Quirk, K., Evans, J. J., and Watson, P. (2007). Using a Paging System in the Rehabilitation of Encephalitic Patients. *Neuropsychological Rehabilitation*, 17(4–5): 567–81.

Evans, J. J., Emslie, H., and Wilson, B. A. (1998). External Cueing Systems in the Rehabilitation of Executive Impairments of Action. *Journal of the International Neuropsychological Society*, 4(4): 399–408.

Evans, J. J., Wilson, B. A., Needham, P., and Brentnall, S. (2003). Who Makes Good Use of Memory Aids? Results of a Survey of People with Acquired Brain Injury. *Journal of the International Neuropsychological Society*, 9(6): 925–35.

Fish, J., Evans, J. J., Nimmo, M., Martin, E., Kersel, D., Bateman, A., and Wilson, B. A. (2007). Rehabilitation of Executive Dysfunction Following Brain Injury: "Content-Free" Cueing Improves Everyday Prospective Memory Performance. *Neuropsychologia*, 45(6): 1318–30.

Fish, J., Manly, T., and Wilson, B. A. (2008a). Long-term Compensatory Treatment of Organizational Deficits in a Patient with Bilateral Frontal Lobe Damage. *Journal of the International Neuropsychological Society*, 14(1): 154–63.

Fish, J., Manly, T., Emslie, H., Evans, J. J., and Wilson, B. A. (2008b). Compensatory Strategies for Acquired Disorders of Memory and Planning: Differential Effects of a Paging System for Patients with Brain Injury of Traumatic Versus Cerebrovascular Aetiology. *Journal of Neurology, Neurosurgery and Psychiatry*, 79(8): 930–35.

Fish, J., Wilson, B. A., and Manly, T. (2010). The Assessment and Rehabilitation of Prospective Memory Problems in People with Neurological Disorders: A Review. *Neuropsychological Rehabilitation*, 20(2): 161–79.

Fleming, J. M., Shum, D., Strong, J., and Lightbody, S. (2005). Prospective Memory Rehabilitation for Adults with Traumatic Brain Injury: A Compensatory Training Programme. *Brain Injury*, 19(1): 1–10.

Gentry, T., Wallace, J., Kvarfordt, C., and Lynch, K. B. (2008). Personal Digital Assistants as Cognitive Aids for Individuals with Severe Traumatic Brain Injury: A Community-Based Trial. *Brain Injury*, 22(1): 19–24.

Giles, G. M. and Shore, M. (1989). The Effectiveness of an Electronic Memory Aid for a Memory-Impaired Adult of Normal Intelligence. *The American Journal of Occupational Therapy*, 43(6): 409–11.

Gillespie, A., Best, C., and O'Neill, B. (2012). Cognitive Function and Assistive Technology for Cognition: A Systematic Review. *Journal of the International Neuropsychological Society*, 18(1): 1–19.

Gillette, Y. and DePompei, R. (2004). The Potential of Electronic Organizers as a Tool in the Cognitive Rehabilitation of Young People. *NeuroRehabilitation*, 19(3): 233–43.

Hasvold, P. and Wootton, R. (2011). Use of Telephone and SMS Reminders to Improve Attendance at Hospital Appointments: A Systematic Review. *Journal of Telemedicine and Telecare*, 17: 358–64.

Hermann, D., Brubaker, B., Yoder, C., Sheets, Y., and Tio, A. (1999). Devices That Remind. In Durso, F. T., Nickerson, R. S., Schvaneveldt, R. W., Dumais, S. T., Lindsay, D. S., and Chi, M. T. H. (eds), *Handbook of Applied Cognition*. New York, NY: John Wiley and Sons.

Hodges, S., Berry, E., and Wood, K. (2011). SenseCam: A Wearable Camera That Stimulates and Rehabilitates Autobiographical Memory. *Memory*, 19(7): 685–96.

Horvath, T., Azman, H., Kennedy, G., and Rutherford, G. (2012). Mobile Phone Text Messaging for Promoting Adherence to Antiretroviral Therapy in Patients with HIV Infection. *Cochrane Database Systematic Reviews*, 3: CD009756.

Jeong, J. M. and Cranney, J. (2009). Motivation, Depression and Naturalistic Time-Based Prospective Remembering. *Memory*, 17(7): 732–41.

Johnson, K., Bamer, A., Yorkston, K., and Amtmann, D. (2009). Use of Cognitive Aids and Other Assistive Technology by Individuals with Multiple Sclerosis. *Disability and Rehabilitation: Assistive Technology*, 4: 1–8.

Kapur, N. and Wilson, B. A. (2009). Compensating for Memory Deficits with Memory Aids. In Wilson, B. A. (ed.), *Memory Rehabilitation: Integrating Theory and Practice*. New York, NY: The Guilford Press.

Kapur, N., Glisky, E. L., and Wilson, B. A. (2004). External Memory Aids and Computers in Memory Rehabilitation. In Baddeley, A. D., Kopelman, M. D., and Wilson, B. A. (eds), *The Essential Handbook of Memory Disorders for Clinicians*. Chichester, UK: John Wiley and Sons.

Kikhia, B., Hallberg, J., Synnes, K., and Sani, Z. (2009). Context-Aware Life-Logging for Persons with Mild Dementia. *Conference Proceedings IEEE Engineering in Medicine and Biology Society*: 6183–6.

Lemoncello, R. and Prideaux, J. (2011). A Randomised Controlled Crossover Trial Evaluating Television Assisted Prompting (TAP) for Adults with Acquired Brain Injury. *Neuropsychological Rehabilitation*, 6: 825–46.

Levinson, R. B. S. (1997). The Planning and Execution Assistant and Trainer. *The Journal of Head Trauma Rehabilitation*, 12(2): 85–91.

Lloyd-Yeates, T. (2013). Alive to New Possibilities. *The Journal of Dementia Care*, 21: 12–13.

LoPresti, E. F., Mihailidis, A., and Kirsch, N. (2004). Assistive Technology for Cognitive Rehabilitation: State of the Art. *Neuropsychological Rehabilitation*, 14(1/2): 5–39.

LoPresti, E. F., Simpson, R. C., Kirsch, N., Schreckenghost, D., and Hayashi, S. (2008). Distributed Cognitive Aid with Scheduling and Interactive Task Guidance. *Journal of Rehabilitation Research and Development*, 45(4): 505–21.

Loveday, C. and Conway, M. A. (2011). Using SenseCam with an Amnesic Patient: Accessing Inaccessible Everyday Memories. *Memory*, 19(7): 697–704.

McDonald, A., Haslam, C., Yates, P., Gurr, B., Leeder, G., and Sayers, A. (2011). Google Calendar: A New Memory Aid to Compensate for Prospective Memory Deficits Following Acquired Brain Injury. *Neuropsychological Rehabilitation*, 21(6): 784–807.

McLellan, D. L. (1991). Functional Recovery and the Principles of Disability Medicine. In Swash, M. and Oxbury, J. (eds), *Clinical Neurology* (pp. 768–90). Edinburgh: Churchill Livingstone.

Martin-Saez, M., Deakins, J., Winson, R., Watson, P., and Wilson, B. A. (2011). A 10-year Follow up of a Paging Service for People with Memory and Planning Problems within a Healthcare System: How do Recent Users Differ from the Original Users? *Neuropsychological Rehabilitation*, 21(6): 769–83.

O'Neill, B., Moran, K., and Gillespie, A. (2010). Scaffolding Rehabilitation Behaviour Using a Voice-Mediated Assistive Technology for Cognition. *Neuropsychological Rehabilitation*, 20(4): 509–27.

Oriani, M., Moniz-Cook, E., Binetti, G., Zanieri, G., Frisoni, G. B., Geroldi, C., De Vreese, L. P., and Zanetti, O. (2003). An Electronic Memory Aid to Support Prospective Memory in Patients in the Early Stages of Alzheimer's Disease: A Pilot Study. *Aging & Mental Health*, 7(1): 22–7.

Pauly-Takacs, K., Moulin, C. J. A., and Estlin, E. J. (2011). SenseCam as a Rehabilitation Tool in a Child with Anterograde Amnesia. *Memory*, 19(7): 705–12.

Pijnenborg, G. H. M., Withaar, F. K., Evans, J. J., Van Den Bosch, R. J., and Brouwer, W. H. (2007). SMS Text Messages as a Prosthetic Aid in the Cognitive Rehabilitation of Schizophrenia. *Rehabilitation Psychology*, 52(2): 236.

Prasad, S. and Anand, R. (2012). Use of Mobile Telephone Short Message Service as a Reminder: The Effect on Patient Attendance. *International Dental Journal*, 62: 21–6.

Savage, K. R. and Svoboda, E. (2013). Long Term Benefits of the Memory-Link Program in a Case of Amnesia. *Clinical Rehabilitation*, 27(6): 521–26.

Shum, D., Fleming, J., Gill, H., Gullo, M. J., and Strong, J. (2011). A Randomized Controlled Trial of Prospective Memory Rehabilitation in Adults with Traumatic Brain Injury. *Journal of Rehabilitation Medicine*, 43(3): 216–23.

Sohlberg, M. M. (2005). External Aids for Management of Memory Impairment. In High, W. M. (ed.), *Rehabilitation for Traumatic Brain Injury*. Oxford, UK: Oxford University Press.

Sohlberg, M. M. and Mateer, C. A. (1989). Training Use of Compensatory Memory Books: A Three Stage Behavioral Approach. *Journal of Clinical and Experimental Neuropsychology*, 11(6): 871–91.

Sohlberg, M. M., Fickas, S., Hung, P.-F., and Fortier, A. (2007a). A Comparison of Four Prompt Modes For Route Finding For Community Travellers With Severe Cognitive Impairments. *Brain Injury*, 21(5): 531–38.

Sohlberg, M. M., Kennedy, M. R. T., Avery, J., Coelho, C., Turkstra, L., and Ylvisaker, M. (2007b). Evidence Based Practice for the Use of External Aids as Memory Rehabilitation Techniques. *Journal of Medical Speech Pathology*, 15(1): xv–li.

Stapleton, S., Adams, M., and Atterton, L. (2007). A Mobile Phone as a Memory Aid for Individuals with Traumatic Brain Injury: A Preliminary Investigation. *Brain Injury*, 21(4): 401–11.

Svoboda, E. and Richards, B. (2009). Compensating for Anterograde Amnesia: A New Training Method That Capitalizes on Emerging Smartphone Technologies. *Journal of the International Neuropsychological Society*, 15(4): 629–38.

Svoboda, E., Richards, B., Polsinelli, A., and Guger, S. (2010). A Theory-Driven Training Programme in the Use of Emerging Commercial Technology: Application to an Adolescent with Severe Memory Impairment. *Neuropsychological Rehabilitation*, 20(4): 562–86.

Svoboda, E., Richards, B., Leach, L., and Mertens, V. (2012). PDA and Smartphone Use by Individuals with Moderate-To-Severe Memory Impairment: Application of a Theory-Driven Training Programme. *Neuropsychological Rehabilitation*, 22(3): 408–27.

Tate, R. L. (2002). Emotional and Social Consequences of Memory Disorders. In Baddeley, A., Kopelman, M. D. K., and Wilson, B. A. (eds), *The Handbook of Memory Disorders* (2nd edition). Chichester, UK: John Wiley and Sons.

Van den Broek, M. D., Downes, J., Johnson, Z., Dayus, B., and Hilton, N. (2000). Evaluation of an Electronic Memory Aid in the Neuropsychological Rehabilitation of Prospective Memory Deficits. *Brain Injury*, 14(5): 455–62.

Van Hulle, A. and Hux, K. (2006). Improvement Patterns Among Survivors of Brain Injury: Three Case Examples Documenting the Effectiveness of Memory Compensation Strategies. *Brain Injury*, 20(1): 101–09.

Vemuri, S. and Bender, W. (2004). Next Generation Memory Aids. *BT Technology Journal*, 22: 125–38.

Wade, T. K. and Troy, J. C. (2001). Mobile Phones as a New Memory Aid: A Preliminary Investigation Using Case Studies. *Brain Injury*, 15(4): 305–20.

Waldron, B., Grimson, J., Carton, S., and Blanco-Campal, A. (2012). Effectiveness of an Unmodified Personal Digital Assistant as a Compensatory Strategy for Prospective Memory Failures in Adults with an ABI. *The Irish Journal of Psychology*, 33: 29–42.

Wild, M. R. (2011). *Organize Your Life Using the iPod Touch: Making Cognitive Connections at Home, School and Work.* Laguna Hills, CA: ID4 the Web.

Wild, M. R. and Schwartz, S. (2009). A Cost Effective Approach to Traumatic Brain Injury Rehabilitation: The Case for a Systematic PDA Curriculum to Help our Servicemembers with TBI. Available at: http://id4theweb.com/TBI%20Rehab%20w_PDA%20white%20paper.pdf (accessed 28 July 2014).

Wilson, B. A. (2009). *Memory Rehabilitation: Integrating Theory and Practice.* New York, NY: The Guilford Press.

Wilson, B. A. and Watson, P. C. (1996). A Practical Framework for Understanding Compensatory Behaviour in People with Organic Memory Impairment. *Memory*, 4(5): 465–86.

Wilson, B. A. and Evans, J. J. (2003). Does Cognitive Rehabilitation Work? Clinical and Economic Considerations and Outcomes. In Prigatano, G. P. and Pliskin, N. (eds), *Clinical Neuropsychology and Cost Outcome Research: A Beginning* (pp. 329–50). Hove, UK: Psychology Press.

Wilson, B. A., Evans, J. J., Emslie, H., and Malinek, V. (1997). Evaluation of NeuroPage: A New Memory Aid. *Journal of Neurology, Neurosurgery and Psychiatry*, 63(1): 113–15.

Wilson, B. A., Emslie, H. C., Quirk, K., and Evans, J. J. (2001). Reducing Everyday Memory and Planning Problems by Means of a Paging System: A Randomised Control Crossover Study. *Journal of Neurology, Neurosurgery and Psychiatry*, 70: 477–82.

Wilson, B. A., Scott, H., Evans, J., and Emslie, H. (2003). Preliminary Report of a NeuroPage Service within a Health Care System. *NeuroRehabilitation*, 18(1): 3–8.

Wilson, B. A., Emslie, H., Quirk, K., Evans, J., and Watson, P. (2005). A Randomized Control Trial to Evaluate a Paging System for People with Traumatic Brain Injury. *Brain Injury*, 19(11): 891–94.

Wilson, B. A., Emslie, H., Evans, J. J., Quirk, K., Watson, P., and Fish, J. (2009). The NeuroPage System for Children and Adolescents with Neurological Deficits. *Developmental NeuroRehabilitation*, 12(6): 421–26.

World Health Organization (2001). *International Classification of Functioning, Disability and Health* (ICF). Geneva, Switzerland: World Health Organization.

Wright, P., Rogers, N., Hall, C., Wilson, B., Evans, J., Emslie, H., and Bartram, C. (2001). Comparison of Pocket-Computer Memory Aids for People with Brain Injury. *Brain Injury*, 15(9): 787–800.

Yamaguchi, T., Foloppe, D., Richard, P., and Allain, P. (2012). A Dual-Modal Virtual Reality Kitchen for Re(learning) of Everyday Cooking Activities in Alzheimer's Disease. *Presence*, 21: 43–57.

Yasuda, K., Misu, T., Beckman, B., Watanabe, O., Ozawa, Y., and Nakamura, T. (2002). Use of an IC Recorder as a Voice Output Memory Aid for Patients with Prospective Memory Impairment. *Neuropsychological Rehabilitation*, 12: 155–66.

4

AFFECT-AWARE ASSISTIVE TECHNOLOGIES

Omar AlZoubi, M. Sazzad Hussain,
and Rafael A. Calvo

Affects are mental and physiological states influencing cognition, learning, communication, decision making, and other important aspects of human experience (Picard, 1997; Tao and Tan, 2005). Daily life of disabled people is not only affected by physical limitations but also by impairments in the ability to think about themselves and impairments in social interaction with other people (Couture *et al.*, 2006; Penn *et al.*, 1995; Pinkham and Penn, 2006; Stickel *et al.*, 2009). Impairment in the skills of affective adaptation/regulation may hinder adjustment to new situations; the learning of new concepts and communication with people around them. These factors may directly influence the person's well-being (Calvo and Peters, 2014; Ryan and Deci, 2000). Deficits in affect regulation thus add to the difficulties arising from congenital or acquired impairments of other mental functions (LoPresti *et al.*, 2008).

Assistive technologies can reduce the effect of these impairments and improve quality of life, creating possibilities for people with special needs to communicate, work, and perform daily activities efficiently and autonomously (Garay *et al.*, 2006). Assistive technology may include software, hardware, or any kind of technology that provides an individual with greater independence. In this chapter, we will refer to the technological tools that augment the emotional functions, thus enabling people with sensory, motor, and cognitive limitations to achieve more independence and perform activities of their choice (e.g. communication, mobility, work, and so on) (Lewis, 2007; Nancy, 2012).

Assistive technologies have progressed through supports for impairments of mobility, vision, hearing, and, latterly, cognition (Konstantinidis, *et al.*, 2009; Moore and Taylor, 2000; Park *et al.*, 2012). However, Garay *et al.* (2006) pointed to a lack of research work on assistive technology for emotion. They described a number of impairments and disorders that may involve affective communication deficits in various stages of affective processing (sensing, expressing, or interpreting affect-relevant signals). They also provided some insights on technologies that can be used to alleviate the lack of affective communication in certain disabilities. According to their definition, Affective Computing aims to capture and process affective information to enhance the communication between the human and the computer, while affective mediation uses an affect-aware computer system as an intermediary to enhance affective communication.

During the 1980s, researchers began to hypothesize about how computer systems could be used for studying emotions, and systematic approaches began in the early 1990s (Calvo and D'Mello, 2010; Scherer, 1993; Turkle, 1984). Studying emotions has received great attention from computer scientists since the late 1990s. Since then, Affective Computing has become a mature discipline with specialized journals (e.g. the *IEEE Transactions on Affective Computing*) and major compilations (Calvo *et al.*, forthcoming). Among the areas of fastest growth is the development of technologies to aid learning and cognitive tasks (Calvo and D'Mello, 2011), in conditions such as autism spectrum disorder (Kaliouby *et al.*, 2006), and, even more generally, in the promotion of psychological well-being (Calvo and Peters, 2014). New input sources, such as eye gaze tracking, speech, facial expression recognition, and even physiological sensors, which act as affect indicators, are being used in affect-aware systems. The large amount of multimodal data available, combined with machine-learning techniques, can be used to develop systems that are able to detect various affective states and provide intelligent responses (Calvo and D'Mello, 2010). While the primary focus of Affective Computing research has been toward human–computer interaction for cognitively intact people (e.g. computer gaming, intelligent tutoring systems, and so on), recent work has aimed to create new assistive technologies that are increasingly reliant on physiological measures of affective processes (Kaliouby *et al.*, 2006). Bringing Affective Computing and assistive technologies research together has significant potential for enhancing affective communication and providing better solutions to assist people with a disability.

Developing systems that can detect affective states from people with disabilities is a complex and challenging task. Researchers in Affective Computing rely on multiple cues or modalities for detecting affects, which include facial expressions, vocal patterns, physiology, and somatic activity. In people with brain impairments, some of these modalities are not always feasible. For example, facial expression or posture is a much less accurate modality in people with muscular dystrophy or chronic pain, because the disease can cause decreased facial expression. Physiological measures, (e.g. heart activity, skin response, respiration pattern, pupil dilation, body temperature) are sometimes more viable options because they can be continuously monitored, are suitable for reflecting inner feelings, and offer a high time resolution (AlZoubi *et al.*, 2011; Picard *et al.*, 2001).

Affective Computing offers enhancements to efforts that address cognitive and affective processing impairments. Robinson and El Kaliouby (2009) argue that affect sensing and expressing technologies can enhance emotion recognition, communication, and regulation in conditions such as autism, anxiety, learning disorders, and visual impairments. In order to build affect-aware assistive technologies, the system needs to be able to detect affects with reasonable accuracy and provide suitable feedback.

In this chapter, we discuss the techniques and modalities used in Affective Computing research. We also review some of the existing work on affect-aware assistive technologies that can provide support to people with various impairments in affective communication.

Affect detection: modalities and techniques

It is the general belief that, in order to give computers the ability to recognize affect, it is necessary to use their vision (i.e. camera) and hearing (e.g. microphone) capabilities for developing the ability to infer affective cues from these and other modalities or sensors. One model that has been used is the categorical model, which postulates that peoples' facial expressions reflect their experiences and feelings (especially the "basic" emotions of happiness, sadness, anger, fear, surprise, and disgust). Inspired by this, in the early 1970s Paul Ekman (1994) started working on facial expressions and found strong evidence that the "basic" emotions (happiness, sadness, anger, fear, surprise, and disgust) are expressed universally. In his research he developed a technique, the Facial Action Coding System (FACS) (Ekman and Friesen, 1978), that defines the human face by a number of Action Units (AUs) and this is the most common technique used for representing the facial expressions in respect to these "basic" emotions. Researchers have been inspired by Ekman's work to analyze facial expressions through image processing techniques (Black and Yacoob, 1995; Essa and Pentland, 1997; Mase, 1991; Otsuka and Ohya, 1997). This approach has shown to be reasonably accurate with the advantage of being non-intrusive and inexpensive since most computers are equipped with webcams (Bartlett et al., 2006; Pantic and Patras, 2006). Other alternative bodily modalities, such as posture and gestures, have also been explored using computer vision-based analysis as part of emotion expression (Calvo and D'Mello, 2010).

The dimensional model is an alternative to the categorical one for representing affect (Russell, 1980). This model describes affects as numerical values of dimensions (valence, activation, and so on) rather than in terms of a small number of categorical, discrete labels (Russell, 2003). The valence dimension measures how humans feel, from positive to negative. The activation or arousal dimension measures the intensity of feelings. Self-reports are used to measure and label emotions by asking the person to rate their feeling either categorically, or numerically using valance-arousal dimensions (Lang et al., 1993). While obtaining accurate self-reports from healthy people is challenging, this is particularly inconvenient for people on the autistic spectrum (Hill et al., 2004; Picard, 2009) given the social, language, and communication difficulties present in this condition. In such cases, we can use the fact that affects can involve more than just the outer behavioral expression but also embodiments, which includes feelings, thoughts, and other internal processes. Physiological measurements have shown to provide useful information about people's inner states and showed to be different from the outer appearance (Picard, 2009). For example, an autistic person can have higher heart rate (Goodwin et al., 2006) or electro-dermal activity (EDA) despite appearing to be calm from the outside (Hirstein et al., 2001).

In the nineteenth century, William James (1884) described emotion as the experience of bodily changes, such as human heart pounding or hands perspiring. Schachter and Singer (Schachter, 1964: Schachter and Singer, 1962) also showed, in experiment, that embodied arousal induced in different situations could trigger different moods. One of the big challenges in emotion theory is whether distinct physiological patterns correlate to certain emotions or dimensions. Despite controversy around some of the results, some physiological correlation of emotions could be identified more frequently than others (Peter and Beale, 2008). Ekman *et al.* (1983) and Winton *et al.* (1984) provided some early findings that showed significant distinctions in autonomic nervous system signals in respect to a small number of emotional states (Picard *et al.*, 2001). It was observed that heart rate can be associated with valence (positive and negative) and skin conductance can be associated with arousal (Lichtenstein *et al.*, 2008). Some other physiological measures are also important for understanding emotions; for example, the diameter of pupil dilation (Herbon *et al.*, 2005) and EMG (electromyography) activities in the zygomatic and corrugator muscles (Lichtenstein *et al.*, 2008) have demonstrated to correlate with valence. Physiological approaches are inspired by the theories of the embodiment of emotion (Calvo and D'Mello, 2010). Several studies have focused on affect detection from physiological signals (e.g. heart activity, skin response, respiration, blood flow, and so on) using machine-learning techniques to identify patterns corresponding to affects (AlZoubi *et al.*, 2011; Calvo and D'Mello, 2010; Healey, 2000; Hussain *et al.*, 2011; Peter *et al.*, 2009; Picard *et al.*, 2001; Wagner *et al.*, 2005; Whang and Lim, 2008). Despite the existing challenges with physiological-based affect detection, such as identifying the right signals and features, detection accuracies, environmental changes, and so forth, the use of physiological measures of valence and arousal hold potential in a variety of applications in the areas of affect, cognition, and behavior.

A variety of modalities can be considered for affect detection (see Table 4.1). Pattern recognition techniques can be used to build affect detectors using information extracted from one or a combination of modalities (Calvo and D'Mello, 2010). The way we interact with each other and interpret affect is naturally multimodal. Humans speak, look, make expressions, and move at the same time as they transition between different affective states. The humans they interact with are constantly interpreting affect from these signals; therefore, using only facial expression, speech, or physiology is not likely to be enough for computer systems to achieve similar accuracy. Combining information from more than one source (i.e. modality) is likely to improve the accuracy of affect detection (D'Mello and Kory, 2012; Pantic and Rothkrantz, 2003). The uncertainties in single modality involve missing features, failure to measure all relevant attributes, and ambiguity (Hall and Llinas, 1997). Therefore, it is advantageous to have multimodal systems where a quantity can be observed and characterized for improved decision making (Sharma *et al.*, 1998). The reader is referred to Calvo *et al.* (forthcoming) for a more in-depth discussion of state-of-the-art Affective Computing and affective detection.

TABLE 4.1 Popular affect detection modalities and description

Modality	Description
Facial expression	Derives facial features using image and video analysis related to emotions
Gesture and posture	Interprets human gesture and posture related to emotional behavior
Emotional speech	Detects emotional states by analyzing speech patterns (pitch variables, speech rate)
Emotional text	Derives high quality information from text related to emotions
Facial electromyogram (EMG)	Expressions from facial muscle activities (e.g. due to smile, frown)
Electrocardiogram (ECG)	Interpretation of the electrical activity of the heart over a period of time. Heart activity related information (e.g. heart-beat variability)
Galvanic skin response (GSR)	Electrical conductance of the skin, which measures the level of sweat in a particular gland. Also known as skin conductivity (SC)
Blood volume pressure (BVP)	The pressure against the walls of blood vessels due to blood flow
Respiration (RESP)	Breathing pattern, inhaling/exhaling rate
Electroencephalogram (EEG)	Brain activity signals

Affective disabilities and affective mediation technologies

Emotional intelligence consists of the ability to recognize, express, and feel emotions, besides the ability to self-regulate these emotions (Picard, 1997). Impairments may occur in one or more of these stages. In this section we present and discuss some of these disabilities, the affective processing impairment associated with it, and the possible affective technologies that could enhance people's affect processing and recognition abilities.

Overcoming sensory impairments

The loss of eyesight or having poor vision can bring with it major difficulties for living a productive life and maintaining effective communication in social settings. It is estimated that nearly 65 percent of the information transmitted during inter-personal communication happens through non–verbal communication cues (Krishna et al., 2010). While speech can contain most of the information, non-verbal cues add to the exchange and interpretation of this verbal information. For example, the puckering of the lip, arms folded, shoulders slumped, eyes averted, or prolonged stare all convey important information about the affective state of an individual. People communicate using facial expressions, voice, body language, and other modalities. Although dependent on the level of impairment, it would be fair to say it would be hard or impossible for someone with a non-correctable visual impairment to see other people's visual affective cues (e.g. facial expression, eye gaze, body language, and gestures). Therefore, communication in this case must take place using other senses. Visual impairment brings difficulties in accomplishing critical tasks that require a certain degree of emotional intelligence (e.g. deception detection). Inability to sense and recognize affective cues from other people can also hinder the ability to emotionally self-regulate. Children with visual disabilities find it especially difficult to learn social skills in development among sighted peers, which can lead to social isolation (Krishna *et al.*, 2010). Most blind and visually impaired individuals can eventually adapt to the lack of visual information and lead a productive lifestyle. However, the path to effective adaptation could be enhanced through the use of assistive aids. Thus, one of the goals of affect-aware systems is to help people with visual impairments sense affective cues and respond to them intelligently (Robinson and El Kaliouby, 2009).

Similarly, hearing disorders such as deafness introduce major communication difficulties. Deaf people are not able to process the explicit emotional message transmitted by speech or the voice intonation associated with it (Garay *et al.*, 2006). Unaided deaf and blind people lose most of the affective information conveyed in these modalities of communication.

A number of technologies have been designed for people with visual and hearing disorders. An interesting assistive technology for visually impaired people has been developed by Krishna *et al.* (2010), the VibroGlove – an interface designed to enhance human–human interpersonal interactions. It can detect and deliver facial expressions of the interacting partner. Vibro-tactors (vibration motors), mounted on the back of the glove provide a means for conveying haptic emoticons that represent the six basic emotions and the neutral expression of the interacting partner. The VibroGlove consists of 14 vibration motors mounted on the back of the fingers, one per phalange. The facial recognition software focuses on detecting affective cues from the mouth area. This information is then used to design spatiotemporal haptic alternates for the six basic emotions plus the neutral expression. They used nine vibrators on the three central fingers to convey the mouth shapes, and effectively the facial expression, to the user. For example, "happy" is represented by a U shaped pattern, "sad" by an inverted U, "surprise" by a circle and neutral by a straight line. They conducted an experiment with one blind participant and 11 sighted, but blindfolded, participants for recognizing the seven emotional expressions. Participants were able to achieve 89 percent recognition rate of emotions indicating the potential of the tool as an assistive aid for the blind.

On the other hand, El Kaliouby and Robinson (2003) reported on an emotional hearing aid that is intended to aid people with autism spectrum disorder (ASD) to recognize emotions. Although people with ASD are the target for this application, the device could also be beneficial for people who are visually impaired. The emotional hearing aid consists of a facial recognition system with software running on a server. Facial expressions of conversational partners can be detected using cameras and sent to a server wirelessly for processing and classifying emotions. The detected emotion is then transferred back to the hearing aid using covert voice in an unobtrusive way. The application is analogous to a hearing aid, which allows people with hearing problems to communicate with the rest of the world.

In a similar fashion, Garay *et al.* (2006) reported on Gestele, an assistive technology designed to provide affective communication for people with speaking disabilities. It is a multimodal affective mediation technology that includes emotional expressivity hints through voice intonation and preconfigured small talk. It also allows message composition using different input options directly or by scanning, depending on user characteristics. This allows someone with speaking disability to hold telephone conversations with others in an effective way. The system can be viewed as a text-to-speech system, where composed messages can be spoken using speech synthesis software. The volume, pitch, and speed used by the system are tuned to reflect users' emotions. The automatic generation of affect within spoken sentences relies on two factors, the emotion, and the style of conversation, which are set by the user. The emotion consists of four values (happiness, sadness, anger, and neutral) and the style of conversation takes on four values (formal, informal, humorous, and aggressive). The system was tested with 25 volunteers to detect the emotion in the speech from direct and synthesized voice generated by the system. Results showed that there were no significant differences in emotion perception for the voice directly heard or heard over the telephone.

Affect-aware technology and mobility impairments

Locked-in syndrome is a severe motor disability that is characterized by inability to produce speech, move limbs, or form facial expressions, even though the person is awake and conscious. This condition may result from a variety of reasons including traumatic brain injury, stroke, and neurological disease. There have been efforts to design assistive technology that can help these people perform certain tasks through brain–computer interface devices (BCI) (Wolpaw *et al.*, 2002). BCI technology aims to compensate for the loss of motor function by enabling the disabled person to communicate through a non-muscular channel. It relies on certain features from the brain activity signals (e.g. mu rhythmic activity of EEG), which can be intentionally controlled by the patient. These signals can then be translated into output commands to control a wheelchair or some computer application (e.g. word spelling application). In addition to controls, there have been efforts to apply BCI techniques to affect detection and biofeedback (Molina *et al.*, 2009). Patients with severe motor disability can benefit the most from this technology, as it can serve as an assessment tool and enable them to communicate with the outside world. An affective BCI could allow the communication and expression of not only content but also affect between the patient and caregiver.

Motor recovery after stroke or traumatic brain injury is a complex process that starts with incapacity to move the affected limb. Stroke survivors can often regain some or all movement over time through training therapies. Mihelj *et al.* (2009) designed an affect-aware system for aiding people with upper extremity motor disabilities.

The system combines an immersive virtual environment coupled with multimodal sensory feedbacks, which are intended to improve neuro-rehabilitation movement training. The movement training significantly improved through immersive multimodal sensory feedback. The feedback loop consisted of detecting patients' activities within the virtual environment so that effects are experienced in a meaningful and purposeful way rather than just a mechanical training. The second aspect of feedback is to reflect back the patient's psychophysiological state into the environment, and use this input to adapt intelligently to their state according to the goals defined by the specific sensory-motor deficit.

Affective computing techniques have also been used in the Emotion and Pain Project. The project proposes an intelligent system to monitor and assess a patient's mood (pain-related) and physical activity. The system presents a module to automatically detect a patient's emotional state, which is then used to provide personalized feedback and support during physical therapy sessions (Singh *et al.*, 2012).

Identifying emotion in others

ASD is a lifelong developmental disability that affects cognitive and socio-emotional skills including social interaction, language acquisition, and imaginative skills. People with ASD focus on parts rather than wholes according to the weak central coherence account model (Happé and Frith, 2006). They often show superior performance on tasks that require focus; however, tasks that require integration of many sensory stimuli or abstract concepts can be difficult for them to accomplish. This can include correctly guessing other people's state of mind in social settings or imagining future states appropriately to plan a task (LoPresti *et al.*, 2008). Difficulty recognizing facial expressions is common in people with ASD, as well as difficulties in emotional vocal recognition (Garay *et al.*, 2006). The social disability of people with ASD is a profound one affecting their capacity for understanding other people, their emotions, and for establishing reciprocal relationships (Scassellati, 2007).

It has been suggested that people with autism benefit from rehearsing different emotional situations repeatedly (Picard, 1997). Thus, it would be beneficial to have computers that would be able to provide such training. Current assistive technology for instruction and communication with autistic children involves the use of visual support systems and the use of social stories, which help them to understand social interactions and situations. Children with autism have shown increased attention and motivation with computer intervention programs as opposed to the traditional student–teacher social skills training (Chen and Bernard-Opitz, 1993).

A growing number of studies have emerged with applications of advanced interactive technologies to address emotional deficits related to autism. These include computer games, virtual reality, social robotics systems, and self-reflecting wearable sensors. Park *et al.* (2012) proposed the use of serious games as an assistive technology to teach emotions to autistic children. The game design framework helps learning and cognitive development processes. The main aim of the games is to assist the children in recognizing facial expressions of emotions using six different modes (recognizing, matching, observing, understanding, generalizing, and mimicking).

One of the basic themes in social robotics is the development of socially assistive robots to help humans with deficient social skills by simulating social interactions. Socially intelligent robotics is a special branch of social assistive robotics that aims to create robots that are capable of having natural social communication abilities (Tapus *et al.*, 2007). Social assistive robots are hypothesized to be able to enhance the quality of life for people with cognitive disabilities and developmental disorders such as ASD. Social robotics technologies generate a high degree of motivation and engagement for people with ASD (Scassellati, 2007). Assistive robots offer a distinctive way to quantify social behavior; these systems offer repeatable, impartial, and measurable description of social responses of an individual that is free of observer's prejudice. Conn *et al.* (2008) described how a social robot was used to detect emotions from autistic children using their physiological response and adapt the behavior accordingly. Their experimental setup consisted of computer-based cognitive tasks and a robot-based basketball game. They were able to achieve 82 percent concordance with therapist rated affect.

Wearable technologies that rely on self-affect sensing and recognition have also been developed, and aim to help increase self-awareness and provide new ways for self-monitoring for people with ASD. Kaliouby *et al.* (2006) described what they call a self-cam, which uses a small video camera worn over the chest to point toward one's face. The camera tracks and analyzes the mental state of its wearer in real time, and communicates this back to him or her visually, or via audio or vibration. Multiple cameras worn by multiple people can communicate with each other allowing the wearers to explore social situations relevant to them. Sarrafzadeh *et al.* (2009) developed a wearable facial expression recognition system that can assist autistic children recognize emotions in others. Their system consisted of a miniature camera, hidden inside a hat worn by the user, and facial expression recognition software. The hat camera was connected wirelessly to a small processing unit placed in the user's pocket. The facial expression recognition component was able to identify emotions and communicated this back to the user through pressure gloves in order to make them aware of this in real time.

Virtual reality environments (VRE) have been used to assist people with ASD. Welch *et al.* (2009) described how VRE can be used to assist in ASD diagnosis and treatment. They suggested a method where a VR system will present realistic social communication tasks, which rely on an avatar telling a story and asking questions to children with ASD while monitoring their physiological responses. The system manipulated the social communication tasks in order to allow understanding of the behavioral components of the children with autism, detect affective states, and respond to them intelligently. They chose to monitor physiological responses because autistic children often have communicative impairments in expressing their affective states using common modalities (facial, verbal, and body language). Virtual reality is envisioned to be a medium well-suited for creating interactive intervention paradigms for skill training in the main areas of impairment (i.e. social interaction, social communication, and imagination), and be able to automate the time-consuming routine behavioral therapy sessions. The system relies on two social parameters; namely, the eye gaze and social proximity of the avatar. These parameters were chosen by the researchers because they play a significant role in social interaction.

Fabri *et al.* (2007) developed a virtual messenger that offers a computer mediated affective communication for people with ASD. The system uses emotionally expressive avatars to allow two spatially separated users to meet virtually. The avatars are capable of displaying the six basic emotions, expressing the users' current emotional state. Users see each other's virtual representation, chat with each other, and express emotions via their animated avatar heads. The authors argue that the tool could be used as an assistive tool allowing people with ASD to communicate more effectively, as they believe the tool offers communication that is simpler and less threatening than its face-to-face equivalent. The direct and active control over interaction may also increase confidence of people who otherwise feel out of control in social situations.

The MIT media lab is actively working on new Affective Computing technologies that are targeted toward people with ASD. Picard (2009) described how a wireless EDA sensor (the Q-Sensor) attached to a wristband can be used for measuring the arousal level of an autistic person. Autistic people may experience a high level of emotional arousal while still looking completely calm; therefore, their physiological responses may be a suitable means for measuring emotional behavior where sensors such as facial and voice may fail. Picard ran an experiment with autistic people equipped with the EDA wristband. The EDA signal was transferred to a computer where it was processed. Their level of arousal was then communicated to others through a graph.

Technologies to reduce anxiety and excessive arousal

Post-traumatic stress disorder (PTSD) is a complex disorder incorporating behavioral, emotional, and cognitive factors. PTSD can arise from a range of situations, such as warfare, natural disaster, vehicular collisions, or interpersonal violence. It is characterized by reoccurring panic and anxiety attacks. People with PTSD may suffer from other particular problems related to emotion regulation, memory and attention, self-perception, and interpersonal relations (Wiederhold and Wiederhold, 2010). Disturbances caused by PTSD can cause significant distress or impairment in social, occupational, or other important areas of functioning (Cooper and Michels, 1981). The two primary symptoms for people suffering from PTSD are re-experiencing or flashbacks and dissociation (Naze and Treur, 2011). Re-experiencing occurs when the patient experiences a strong emotional state similar to that felt during the traumatic event, often associated with visual flashbacks and physical distress. Dissociation refers to the experience of emotional withdrawal on account of the emotional load triggered by a stimulus, often including a loss of body perception or the so-called out-of-body experience.

Affective processing theory suggests that, in order to decrease anxiety associated with PTSD, anxiety must first be elicited by triggering it through simulating or imaging real-life scenarios (Wiederhold and Wiederhold, 2010). However, this approach carries many undesired side effects for patients and clinicians, such as high levels of emotional distress for both patients and clinicians. Effective treatments to calm anxiety include relaxation training, realistic exposure therapy, and imaginal exposure therapy. Real-life exposure therapy may not be feasible and imaginal exposure therapy may not elicit the desired level of anxiety. Virtual reality exposure treatment (VRET) holds great promise for people with PTSD as it can offer a personalized, private treatment environment (Krijn et al., 2004). A person suffering from PTSD can practice the cognitive skills necessary to overcome the trauma during exposure to a virtual trauma situation in a controllable and personalized manner. VRET has many other advantages over traditional exposure approaches that include maintaining patients' confidentiality, flexibility, cost effectiveness, and safety (Wiederhold and Wiederhold, 2010). In addition, physiological feedback can provide patients with a sense of control by being aware of their physiological reactions during stress or relaxation. This may give them the ability to self-monitor and control bodily reactions during times of stress. In one case study, VRET was combined with two other methods (relaxation and imaginary exposure) to treat a Vietnam veteran for fourteen 90-minute sessions over six weeks. The participant showed a 34 percent decrease on his clinically rated PTSD (Rothbaum et al., 1999). The single case study has yet to be replicated in larger well-controlled studies, but remains promising.

There is other ongoing work on tools that use affect recognition, sensor technologies, and virtual reality to support people with PTSD. For example, Broek (2011) proposed Computer-Aided Diagnosis (CAD), which utilizes speech signals to aid in the treatment PTSD. CAD is envisioned to enable objective, unobtrusive stress measurements that can be used for stress management and treatment. Likewise, Pedersen et al. (2012) designed an adaptive virtual reality system to aid in treatment of PTSD. The system integrates three therapeutic approaches (relaxation training, stress inoculation training, and exposure therapy) in one multimodal treatment tool. They suggested that adaptive and goal-oriented VR-therapy tools can make psychological therapy more engaging and more effective in treating debilitating anxiety disorders.

Technologies that aim to increase awareness of heart rate variability, a physiological marker for the experience of negative emotional states such as stress and anxiety (Karavidas et al., 2007), depressed mood (Carney et al., 2001), and anger (Denson et al., 2011), have led to some evidence of effectiveness in aiding emotional regulation. Disturbances of each of these emotional states are prevalent psychopathologies after brain injury and the relationship between lowered heart rate variability and anger (Denson et al., 2011) indicates the potential of heart rate biofeedback interventions to address agitation, irritability, and interpersonal problems.

Heart rate variability (HRV) is defined as the amount of fluctuation from the mean heart rate and represents the interaction between sympathetic and parasympathetic influences on the heart. Higher HRV is associated with better physical and mental health (Rechlin et al., 1994). A small number of studies have suggested that biofeedback with instruction to engage in slow diaphragmatic breathing can increase HRV and reduce symptoms in patients with somatization difficulties (Hassett *et al.*, 2007) and depression (Karavidas *et al.*, 2007).

Kim *et al.* (2013) explored whether HRV biofeedback improved emotional regulation and problem-solving ability in patients with moderate to severe brain injury. While the study confirmed an association between an individual's performance and their emotional control, they did not demonstrate significant improvement in their sample. O'Neill and Findlay (2014) showed that HRV biofeedback using the emWave system reduced aggressive challenging behavior in two case studies with people with severe brain injury.

Affect-aware technologies and learning

Students with intellectual disabilities are twice as likely to drop out of school as non-disabled students, and the highest drop-out rate is among students with emotional and behavioral disorders (Dugan *et al.*, 2007). Students who have an emotional or behavioral disorder are more likely to have academic difficulties in reading, writing, and mathematics, typifying specific learning disabilities (Edyburn, 2006).

Affect-aware learning systems promise to provide personalized, adaptive, and more effective technology-mediated learning to people with disabilities. Cristescu (2008) advocates for designing educational systems that offer universal access and take into account emotional aspects of disabled people, such as providing affective feedback to increase learning motivation. Education, therefore, might also focus on the learning of social communication skills (Fabri *et al.*, 2007).

Conclusion

Affect-aware assistive technologies are being developed as a new area of research that has the potential to help people with a variety of cognitive impairments. There is a consensus that integrating affective intelligence in assistive technologies research is an essential step to enhance the lives of individuals with affective impairments. People with different sorts of affective disabilities (e.g. ASD, PTSD) could use these affect-aware assistive aids to enhance emotion recognition, communication, and self-regulation.

This chapter has presented implementations of affect-aware systems and demonstrated how they can address the deficits in different stages of affective processing (sensing, expressing, and interpretation). The various disabilities described may exhibit different degrees of impairment of emotional functioning. Therefore, affect-aware technologies may help train disabled people to improve their cognitive functioning and, in other cases, provide a means of assistance to lead a normal and productive life.

Despite the progress made in Affective Computing research, the implementation of an adaptive, multimodal, robust system with sufficient reliability for everyday use remains a distant aim. Challenges still exist in the intrusive nature of physiological sensors, noise artifacts in data, and gathering realistic data to train pattern recognition algorithms. Most of the work is conducted in lab settings and replicating research in more realistic environments is often challenging. Sensors that measure physiological and behavioral responses need to be wearable, light, and portable. Contemporary video-based sensors (e.g. Microsoft Kinect, remote eye trackers) offer remote sensing of physiological features with the help of advanced signal processing and algorithm design. Advances in sensor technologies, wearable devices, and algorithm design will help devise more sophisticated and practical affect-aware technologies.

Affective Computing research will continue to provide improved solutions for affect sensing and detection, and enhance the practicality of affect-aware systems. The field will then likely progress to more robust clinical trials than those realized thus far. This effort will provide assistive technologies with information (e.g. modality and features), tools (e.g. sensors and devices), and techniques (e.g. pattern recognition algorithms) for building and perfecting systems that aim to help people with cognitive impairment improve their ability to recognize, feel, and express emotion.

References

AlZoubi, O., Hussain, M. S., D'Mello, S., and Calvo, R. A. (2011). Affective Modeling from Multichannel Physiology: Analysis of Day Differences. In S. D'Mello, A. Graesser, B. Schuller, and J.-C. Martin (eds), *Proceedings of the 4th International Conference on Affective Computing and Intelligent Interaction,* Memphis, TN (Vol. 6974, pp. 4–13). Berlin, Germany: Springer-Verlag.

Bartlett, M. S., Littlewort, G., Frank, M., Lainscsek, C., Fasel, I., and Movellan, J. (2006). Fully Automatic Facial Action Recognition in Spontaneous Behavior. Paper presented at the *7th International Conference on Automatic Face and Gesture Recognition* (FGR06), April 02–06, Southampton, UK.

Black, M. J. and Yacoob, Y. (1995). Tracking and Recognizing Rigid and non-Rigid Facial Motions Using Local Parametric Models of Image Motion. Paper presented at the *Fifth International Conference on Computer Vision,* June 20–23, Massachusetts, USA.

Broek, E. L. v. d. (2011). *Affective Signal Processing (ASP): Unraveling the Mystery of Emotions.* PhD Thesis. University of Twente, Enschede, the Netherlands. Available at: http://doc.utwente.nl/78025/ (accessed 26 September 2014).

Calvo, R. A. and D'Mello, S. (2010). Affect Detection: An Interdisciplinary Review of Models, Methods and their Applications. *IEEE Transactions on Affective Computing,* 1(1): 18–37.

Calvo, R. A. and D'Mello, S. (2011). *New Perspectives on Affect and Learning Technologies* (Vol. 3). New York, NY: Springer.

Calvo, R. A. and Peters, D. (2014). *Positive Computing: Technology for a Better World.* Cambridge, MA: MIT Press.

Calvo, R. A., D'Mello, S. K., Gratch, J., and Kappas, A. E. (forthcoming). *Handbook of Affective Computing.* Oxford, UK: Oxford University Press.

Carney, R. M., Blumenthal, J. A., Stein, P. K., Watkins, L., Catellier, D., Berkman, L. F., and Freedland, K. E. (2001). Depression, Heart Rate Variability and Acute Myocardial Infarction. *Circulation,* 104(17): 2024–28.

Chen, S. H. A. and Bernard-Opitz, V. (1993). Comparison of Personal and Computer-Assisted Instruction for Children with Autism. *Mental Retardation,* 31: 368–76.

Conn, K., Liu, C., Sarkar, N., Stone, W., and Warren, Z. (2008). Towards Affect-Sensitive Assistive Intervention Technologies for Children with Autism. In J. Or (ed.), *Affective Computing: Focus on Emotion Expression, Synthesis and Recognition* (pp. 365–90). Vienna, Austria: I-Tech Education and Publishing.

Cooper, A. M. and Michels, R. (1981). Diagnostic and Statistical Manual of Mental Disorders. *American Journal of Psychiatry*, 138(1): 128–29.

Couture, S. M., Penn, D. L., and Roberts, D. L. (2006). The Functional Significance of Social Cognition in Schizophrenia: A Review. *Schizophrenia Bulletin*, 32(Suppl. 1): S44–63.

Cristescu, I. (2008). Emotions in Human-Computer Interaction: The Role of Non-verbal Behavior in Interactive Systems. *Revista Informatica Economicănr*, 2(46): 110–16.

D'Mello, S. and Kory, J. (2012). Consistent but Modest: A Meta-analysis on Unimodal and Multimodal Affect Detection Accuracies from 30 Studies. Paper presented at the *14th ACM International Conference on Multimodal Interaction*, Oct. 22–26, Santa Monica, CA.

Denson, T. F., Grisham, J. R., and Moulds, M. L. (2011). Cognitive Reappraisal Increases Heart Rate Variability in Response to an Anger Provocation. *Motivation and Emotion*, 35(1): 14–22.

Dugan, J. J., Cobb, R. B., and Alworth, M. (2007). *The Effects of Technology-Based Interventions on Academic Outcomes for Youth with Disabilities*. Kalamazoo, MI: National Secondary Transition Technical Assistance Center, Western Michigan University.

Edyburn, D. L. (2006). Assistive Technology and Mild Disabilities. *Special Education Technology Practice*, 8(4): 18–28.

Ekman, P. (1994). Strong Evidence for Universals in Facial Expressions: A Reply to Russell's Mistaken Critique. *Psychological Bulletin*, 115(2): 268–87.

Ekman, P. and Friesen, W. (1978). *Facial Action Coding System: A Technique for the Measurement of Facial Movement*. Palo Alto, CA: Consulting Psychologists Press.

Ekman, P., Levenson, R. W., and Friesen, W. V. (1983). Autonomic Nervous System Activity Distinguishes Among Emotions. *Science*, 221(4616): 1208–10.

El Kaliouby, R. and Robinson, P. (2003). The Emotional Hearing Aid: An Assistive Tool for Autism. In C. Stephanidis (ed.), *Proceedings of the Tenth International Conference on Human-Computer Interaction*, June 22–7, Crete, Greece (Vol. 4, pp. 68–72).

Essa, I. A. and Pentland, A. P. (1997). Coding, Analysis, Interpretation and Recognition of Facial Expressions. *IEEE Transactions on Pattern Analysis and Machine Intelligence*, 19(7): 757–63.

Fabri, M., Elzouki, S. Y. A., and Moore, D. (2007). Emotionally Expressive Avatars for Chatting, Learning and Therapeutic Intervention Human–Computer Interaction. *HCI Intelligent Multimodal Interaction Environments* (pp. 275–85). New York, NY: Springer.

Garay, N., Cearreta, I., López, J. M., and Fajardo, I. (2006). Assistive Technology and Affective Mediation. *Human Technology: An Interdisciplinary Journal on Humans in ICT Environments*, 2(1): 55–83.

Goodwin, M. S., Groden, J., Velicer, W. F., Lipsitt, L. P., Baron, M. G., Hofmann, S. G., and Groden, G. (2006). Cardiovascular Arousal in Individuals with Autism. *Focus on Autism and Other Developmental Disabilities*, 21(2): 100–23.

Hall, D. L. and Llinas, J. (1997). An Introduction to Multisensor Data Fusion. *Proceedings of the IEEE*, 85(1): 6–23.

Happé, F. and Frith, U. (2006). The Weak Coherence Account: Detail-Focused Cognitive Style in Autism Spectrum Disorders. *Journal of Autism and Developmental Disorders*, 36(1): 5–25.

Hassett, A. L., Radvanski, D. C., Vaschillo, E. G., Vaschillo, B., Sigal, L. H., Karavidas, M. K., and Lehrer, P. M. (2007). A Pilot Study of the Efficacy of Heart Rate Variability (HRV) Biofeedback in Patients with Fibromyalgia. *Applied Psychophysiology and Biofeedback*, 32(1): 1–10.

Healey, J. A. (2000). *Wearable and Automotive Systems for Affect Recognition from Physiology*, PhD thesis. Cambridge, MA: Massachusetts Institute of Technology.

Herbon, A., Peter, C., Markert, L., Van Der Meer, E., and Voskamp, J. (2005). Emotion Studies in HCI: A New Approach. Paper presented at the *11th International Conference on Human-Computer Interaction*, July 22–27, Las Vegas, NV.

Hill, E., Berthoz, S., and Frith, U. (2004). Brief Report: Cognitive Processing of Own Emotions in Individuals with Autistic Spectrum Disorder and in Their Relatives. *Journal of Autism and Developmental Disorders*, 34(2): 229–35.

Hirstein, W., Iversen, P., and Ramachandran, V. S. (2001). Autonomic Responses of Autistic Children to People and Objects. *Proceedings of the Royal Society of London. Series B: Biological Sciences*, 268(1479):1883–88.

Hussain, M. S., AlZoubi, O., Calvo, R. A., and D'Mello, S. (2011). Affect Detection from Multichannel Physiology during Learning Sessions with AutoTutor. In B. Gautam, B. Susan, K. Judy, and M. Antonija (eds), *Proceedings of the 15th International Conference on Artificial Intelligence in Education* (AIED), Auckland, New Zealand, LNAI (Vol. 6738, pp. 131–38). Berlin, Germany: Springer.

James, W. (1884). What is Emotion? *Mind*, 9(34): 188–205.

Kaliouby, R., Picard, R., and Baron-Cohen, S. (2006). Affective Computing and Autism. *Annals of the New York Academy of Sciences*, 1093(1): 228–48.

Karavidas, M. K., Lehrer, P. M., Vaschillo, E., Vaschillo, B., Marin, H., Buyske, S., and Hassett, A. (2007). Preliminary Results of an Open Label Study of Heart Rate Variability Biofeedback for the Treatment of Major Depression. *Applied Psychophysiology and Biofeedback*, 32(1): 19–30.

Kim, S., Zemon, V., Cavallo, M. M., Rath, J. F., McCraty, R., and Foley, F. W. (2013). Heart Rate Variability Biofeedback, Executive Functioning and Chronic Brain Injury. *Brain Injury*, 27(2): 209–22.

Konstantinidis, E. I., Hitoglou-Antoniadou, M., Luneski, A., Bamidis, P. D., and Nikolaidou, M. M. (2009). Using Affective Avatars and Rich Multimedia Content for Education of Children with Autism. Paper presented at the *2nd International Conference on Pervasive Technologies Related to Assistive Environments*, Corfu, Greece.

Krijn, M., Emmelkamp, P. M., Olafsson, R. P., and Biemond, R. (2004). Virtual Reality Exposure Therapy of Anxiety Disorders: A Review. *Clinical Psychology Review*, 24(3): 259–81.

Krishna, S., Bala, S., McDaniel, T., McGuire, S., and Panchanathan, S. (2010). VibroGlove: An Assistive Technology Aid for Conveying Facial Expressions. Paper presented at the *CHI'10 Extended Abstracts on Human Factors in Computing Systems*, May 5–10, Austin, Texas. Available at: http://dl.acm.org/citation.cfm?id=1753846 (accessed 26 September 2014).

Lang, P. J., Greenwald, M. K., Bradley, M. M., and Hamm, A. O. (1993). Looking at Pictures: Affective, Facial, Visceral and Behavioral Reactions. *Psychophysiology*, 30(3): 261–73.

Lewis, C. (2007). Simplicity in Cognitive Assistive Technology: A Framework and Agenda for Research. *Universal Access in the Information Society*, 5(4): 351–61.

Lichtenstein, A., Oehme, A., Kupschick, S., and Jürgensohn, T. (2008). Comparing Two Emotion Models for Deriving Affective States from Physiological Data. In C. Peter and R. Beale (eds), *Affect and Emotion in Human–Computer Interaction*, LNCS (Vol. 4868, pp. 35–50). Berlin, Germany: Springer.

LoPresti, E. F., Bodine, C., and Lewis, C. (2008). Assistive Technology for Cognition [Understanding the Needs of Persons with Disabilities]. *Engineering in Medicine and Biology Magazine*, 27(2): 29–39.

Mase, K. (1991). Recognition of Facial Expression from Optical Flow. *IEICE Transactions*, E74(10): 3474–83.

Mihelj, M., Novak, D., and Munih, M. (2009). Emotion-Aware System for Upper Extremity Rehabilitation. Paper presented at the *Virtual Rehabilitation International Conference*, June 29–July 02, Haifa, Israel.

Molina, G. G., Tsoneva, T., and Nijholt, A. (2009). Emotional Brain–Computer Interfaces. Paper presented at the *Affective Computing and Intelligent Interaction and Workshops*, ACII 2.009, September 10–12, Amsterdam, the Netherlands. Available at: http://acii2009.fyper.com/ (accessed 26 September 2014).

Moore, D. and Taylor, J. (2000). Interactive Multimedia Systems for Students with Autism. *Journal of Educational Media*, 25(3): 169–77.

Nancy, A. A. (2012). Deployment of Assistive Technology in the Emotional Hearing Aid for Children with Autism. *International Journal of Research in Communication Technologies*, 1(1): 9–12.

Naze, S. and Treur, J. (2011). A Computational Agent Model for Post-Traumatic Stress Disorders (pp. 249–61). In A. V. Samsonovich and K. R. Jóhannsdóttir (eds), *Biologically Inspired Cognitive Architectures BICA 2011: Proceedings of the Second Annual Meeting of the BICA Society*. Amsterdam: IOS Press.

O'Neill, B. and Findlay, G. (2014). Single Case Methodology in Neurobehavioural Rehabilitation: Preliminary Findings on Biofeedback in the Treatment of Challenging Behaviour. *Neuropsychological Rehabilitation*, 24(4): 365–81.

Otsuka, T. and Ohya, J. (1997). Recognizing Multiple Persons' Facial Expressions using HMM Based on Automatic Extraction of Significant Frames from Image Sequences. Paper presented at the *IEEE International Conference on Image Processing*, Oct. 20–29, Washington, DC.

Pantic, M. and Rothkrantz, L. J. M. (2003). Toward an Affect-Sensitive Multimodal Human-Computer Interaction. *Proceedings of the IEEE*, 91(9): 1370–90.

Pantic, M. and Patras, I. (2006). Dynamics of Facial Expression: Recognition of Facial Actions and their Temporal Segments from Face Profile Image Sequences. *IEEE Transactions on Systems, Man and Cybernetics*, Part B, 36(2):433–49.

Park, J. H., Abirached, B., and Zhang, Y. (2012). A Framework for Designing Assistive Technologies for Teaching Children with ASDs Emotions. Paper presented at the *CHI'12 Extended Abstracts on Human Factors in Computing Systems*, May 5–10, Austin, Texas. Available at: http://dl.acm.org/citation.cfm?id=2212776 (accessed 26 September 2014).

Pedersen, C. H., Khaled, R., and Yannakakis, G. N. (2012). Ethical Considerations in Designing Adaptive Persuasive Games (pp. 13–16). In E. L. Ragnemalm and M. Bång (eds), *Proceedings of the 7th International Conference on Persuasive Technology, PERSUASIVE 2012*. Linköping, Sweden: Linköping University Electronic Press.

Penn, D. L., Mueser, K. T., Spaulding, W., Hope, D. A., and Reed, D. (1995). Information Processing and Social Competence in Chronic Schizophrenia. *Schizophrenia Bulletin*, 21(2): 269–81.

Peter, C. and Beale, R. (2008). *Affect and Emotion in Human–Computer Interaction: From Theory to Applications* (Vol. 4868). New York, NY: Springer.

Peter, C., Ebert, E., and Beikirch, H. (2009). Physiological Sensing for Affective Computing. In J. Tao and T. Tan (eds), *Affective Information Processing* (pp. 293–310). New York, NY: Springer-Verlag.

Picard, R. W. (1997). *Affective Computing*. Cambridge, MA: MIT Press.

Picard, R. W. (2009). Future Affective Technology for Autism and Emotion Communication. *Philosophical Transactions of the Royal Society B: Biological Sciences*, 364(1535): 3575–84.

Picard, R. W., Vyzas, E., and Healey, J. (2001). Toward Machine Emotional Intelligence: Analysis of Affective Physiological State. *IEEE Transactions on Pattern Analysis and Machine Intelligence*, 23(10): 1175–91.

Pinkham, A. E. and Penn, D. L. (2006). Neurocognitive and Social Cognitive Predictors of Interpersonal Skill in Schizophrenia. *Psychiatry Research*, 143(2-3): 167–78.

Rechlin, T., Weis, M., Spitzer, A., and Kaschka, W. P. (1994). Are Affective Disorders Associated with Alterations of Heart Rate Variability? *Journal of Affective Disorders*, 32(4): 271–75.

Robinson, P. and El Kaliouby, R. (2009). Computation of Emotions in Man and Machines. *Philosophical Transactions of the Royal Society B: Biological Sciences*, 364(1535): 3441–47.

Rothbaum, B. O., Hodges, L., Alarcon, R., Ready, D., Shahar, F., Graap, K., and Wills, B. (1999). Virtual Reality Exposure Therapy for PTSD Vietnam Veterans: A Case Study. *Journal of Traumatic Stress*, 12(2): 263–71.

Russell, J. A. (1980). A Circumplex Model of Affect. *Journal of Personality and Social Psychology*, 39(6): 1161–78.

Russell, J. A. (2003). Core Affect and the Psychological Construction of Emotion. *Psychological Review*, 110(1): 145–72.

Ryan, R. M. and Deci, E. L. (2000). Self-determination Theory and the Facilitation of Intrinsic Motivation, Social Development and Well-being. *The American Psychologist*, 55(1): 68–78.

Sarrafzadeh, A., Shanbehzadeh, J., Dadgostar, F., Fan, C., and Alexander, S. (2009). Assisting the Autistic with Real-Time Facial Expression Recognition. Paper presented at the *International Conference on Innovations in Information Technology*, Dec. 15–17, Al Ain, UAE.

Scassellati, B. (2007). How Social Robots will Help Us to Diagnose, Treat and Understand Autism. *Robotics Research* (pp. 552–63). New York, NY: Springer.

Schachter, S. (1964). The Interaction of Cognitive and Physiological Determinants of Emotional State. *Advances in Experimental Social Psychology*, 1: 49–80.

Schachter, S. and Singer, J. E. (1962). Cognitive, Social and Physiological Determinants of Emotional State. *Psychological Review*, 69(5): 379–99.

Scherer, K. R. (1993). Studying the Emotion-Antecedent Appraisal Process: An Expert System Approach. *Cognition & Emotion*, 7(3-4): 325–55.

Sharma, R., Pavlovic, V. I., and Huang, T. S. (1998). Toward Multimodal Human–Computer Interface. *Proceedings of the IEEE*, 86(5): 853–69.

Singh, A., Swann-Sternberg, T., Bianchi-Berthouze, N., CdeC Williams, A., Pantic, M., and Watson, P. (2012). Emotion and Pain: Interactive Technology to Motivate Physical Activity in People with Chronic Pain. Paper presented at the *CHI 2012 Workshop: Interaction Design and Emotional Wellbeing: 30th ACM Conference on Human Factors in Computing Systems*, May 05–10, Austin, TX.

Stickel, C., Ebner, M., Steinbach-Nordmann, S., Searle, G., and Holzinger, A. (2009). Emotion Detection: Application of the Valence Arousal Space for Rapid Biological Usability Testing to Enhance Universal Access. In C. Stephanidis (ed.), *Universal Access in Human–Computer Interaction. Addressing Diversity* (Vol. 5614, pp. 615–24). New York, NY: Springer.

Tao, J. H. and Tan, T. N. (2005). Affective Computing: A Review. Paper presented at the *First International Conference on Affective Computing and Intelligent Interaction*, Oct. 22–24, Beijing, China.

Tapus, A., Mataric, M. J., and Scassellati, B. (2007). Socially Assistive Robotics. *IEEE Robotics and Automation Magazine*, 14(1): 35.

Turkle, S. (1984). *The Second Self: Computers and the Human Spirit* (Twentieth Anniversary Edition). New York, NY: Simon & Schuster.

Wagner, J., Kim, J., and Andre, E. (2005). From Physiological Signals to Emotions: Implementing and Comparing Selected Methods for Feature Extraction and Classification. Paper presented at the *IEEE International Conference on Multimedia and Expo*, July 06–08, Amsterdam, the Netherlands.

Welch, K. C., Lahiri, U., Liu, C., Weller, R., Sarkar, N., and Warren, Z. (2009). An Affect-Sensitive Social Interaction Paradigm Utilizing Virtual Reality Environments for Autism Intervention Human–Computer Interaction. *Ambient, Ubiquitous and Intelligent Interaction* (pp. 703–12). New York, NY: Springer.

Whang, M. and Lim, J. (2008). A Physiological Approach to Affective Computing. In J. Or (ed.), *Affective Computing: Focus on Emotion Expression, Synthesis, and Recognition* (pp. 310–18). Vienna, Austria: I-Tech Education and Publishing.

Wiederhold, B. K. and Wiederhold, M. D. (2010). Virtual Reality Treatment of Post-traumatic Stress Disorder due to Motor Vehicle Accident. *CyberPsychology, Behavior and Social Networking*, 13(1): 21–7.

Winton, W. M., Putnam, L. E., and Krauss, R. M. (1984). Facial and Autonomic Manifestations of the Dimensional Structure of Emotion. *Journal of Experimental Social Psychology*, 20(3): 195–216.

Wolpaw, J., Birbaumer, N., McFarland, D., Pfurtscheller, G., and Vaughan, T. (2002). Brain–Computer Interfaces for Communication and Control. *Clinical Neurophysiology*, 113: 767–91.

5

ASSISTIVE TECHNOLOGY FOR DISORDERS OF VISUAL PERCEPTION

Andrew Worthington and Jeremi Sudol

We live in a visual world where our interactions with objects, people, and the environment are primarily mediated by our sense of sight. The brain devotes greater resources to processing visual information than to data from other sensory modalities and this makes vision uniquely vulnerable to disruption from illness or injury. Adults used to normal vision can be severely restricted in their independence following even a modest loss of visual function which can occur following normal ageing, trauma, or disease. Evidence suggests that the problem is increasing. The World Health Organization estimated that there were 161 million people worldwide living with visual impairment in 2002 (Resnikoff *et al.*, 2004) whereas a more recent estimate puts this figure at 285 million, of whom 246 million have a form of low-vision impairment (WHO, 2012). Simple optical devices can be very effective in improving ocular visual problems, but amongst the 14 million visual impairments in the US, for example, 3 million cannot be corrected by contact lenses or spectacles (Vitale *et al.*, 2006).

The true prevalence of visual disorders is undoubtedly far higher than is suggested. Epidemiological surveys generally exclude other forms of "higher" visual dysfunction resulting from neurological disorders such as stroke or dementia, conditions likely to increase as the population ages. A UK multi-center study of stroke survivors (Rowe *et al.*, 2009) reported significant rates of eye-movement disorders (68 percent), field defects (49 percent), low vision (26.5 percent), and perceptual disorders (20.5 percent). Overall, 92 percent had some form of visual impairment when assessed within one month of stroke. Friedman and Leong (1992) reported a perceptual impairment rate of 86 percent in acute stroke, with 64 percent continuing to show signs of impairment after three months. Unless they resolve spontaneously, these visual disorders can cause considerable long-term disability, but are not amenable to conventional methods of correcting eyesight and require innovative technological solutions that are only now starting to be explored.

Visual perceptual processing

In cognitive rehabilitation, having a model of the function or system to be treated provides the basis for a more rational and systematic approach to intervention. Following Marr's (1982) seminal work, most current models of visual perception assume that different components of the visual system are functionally distinct but interact to provide a coherent visual experience. It follows that these separable components can break down selectively. This approach underpinned the cognitive neuropsychological approach to rehabilitation. Thus, Humphreys and Riddoch (1994a) stated: "we believe it is necessary to specify the processes normally subserving visual perception, because it is only by generating such a normal framework that we can understand how vision can break down. We can then go on to use the framework to help the design and evaluation of rehabilitation programs for vision" (1994a: 40).

Essentially, the visual system first has to identify clusters of features that the brain can recognize as objects. The occipital lobes contain highly specialized regions for analyzing specific attributes such as size, shape, color, orientation, depth, and movement. Two distinct pathways then project from the occipital lobes to the parietal and temporal lobes, respectively (Ungerleider and Mishkin, 1982). A ventral pathway from the occipital to the temporal region, sometimes called the "what" pathway, is believed to be responsible for identifying objects. Another pathway streams information dorsally to the (mostly) right parietal region where features are grouped together to make "figure-ground" discriminations and differentiate between objects. Having an integrated perception of an object allows us to identify where an object is from different viewpoints and to calculate relative position. Thus, it has been labeled the "where" pathway, but it also mediates how we interact with objects, suggesting it may be better considered as subserving a "how" function (Milner and Goodale, 1995).

Approaches to the rehabilitation of visual disorders

Unfortunately, the impairment-based approach of cognitive neuropsychological rehabilitation has had limited impact on clinical practice, particularly for visual disorders. In many ways, we have advanced little since Poppelreuter's pioneering work with soldiers injured in the First World War (Poppelreuter, 1917/1990). Efforts to ameliorate visual disorders have remained largely atheoretical and limited in effectiveness, such as the potential of intensive stimulation to improve early-stage visual processing around the margins of hemianopic visual fields (Zihl and von Cramon, 1979; Balliet et al., 1985). Gains have tended to be short-lived and limited to stimulated areas (e.g. Schuett et al., 2012). Hence, in the second edition of his monograph on visual rehabilitation, Zihl (2011) revised his initial enthusiasm for repetitive practice to recommend compensatory approaches as the most appropriate form of intervention in most cases.

Disorders of visual perception

Appreciation of the potential benefits of new technologies for improving visual function can only really be achieved with an understanding of some of the more common and debilitating visual disorders (see Worthington and Riddoch (2008) for a comprehensive overview). The basic premise is that visual disorders can be understood in terms of separable processes and, while the relative contribution of higher-order and lower-order processing continues to excite debate, each can be selectively impaired, though damage in one region can disrupt processing elsewhere.

Disorders of vision

Visual status needs to be considered in any perceptual assessment. This includes both the optical/oculomotor apparatus and the optic tracts. Visual disturbances are commonplace in neurological conditions and current remedial measures, although low-tech, have implications for how more sophisticated tools and devices could be developed. Evidence that selective patching can reduce diplopia without compromising peripheral vision or stereoscopic perception (Politzer, 1996) suggests that it may be possible to produce a similar effect with a contact lens, or even perhaps electronically to "knock-out" information from a portion of the visual field without the need for obtrusive glasses. Light-filtering lenses alleviate the problems of photophobia (Jackowski et al., 1996), but tend to be simple filters only suited to certain environments rather than a dynamic sensitive lens that could be incorporated into hi-tech glasses and goggles. Similar developments could exploit the benefits of current prism lenses to redirect light so that the fixation object is imaged onto the fovea of both eyes, thus reducing double vision and field loss (Rossi et al.,1990). Scanning training has been shown to be linked to increases in visual search field, improved reading speed, and reduced reading errors. Thus, although the evidence is limited, a systematic review recommended that compensatory scanning training was marginally more effective than visual restorative therapy (Bouwmeester et al., 2007). The necessarily repetitive nature, and the need for accurate measurement of scanning, lends itself extremely well to technological innovation. For example, game-based software would provide a fun, motivating training platform that could be customized for the user. Unobtrusive eye-movement trackers that could be worn around the house would provide accurate feedback, not just on training efficacy, but also on generalization to real-world activities. This information could easily be downloaded for reports or sent to therapists for monitoring.

The fact that early-stage deficits can disrupt perception has led some to suggest a hierarchical "bottom-up" model of intervention. Thus, Warren (1993) advocated that basic skills such as oculomotor control, visual fields, and acuity should take precedence, to be built upon with work targeting higher-level complex processing. This has intuitive appeal, but visual processing is not a linear sequence of stages whereby a lower-order deficit inevitably leads to one higher up the system. An illustrative example is DF, a widely studied patient in this field, who was still able to carry out visually-guided actions like reaching for objects and shaking hands despite difficulty completing simple visual tests like perceiving form and line orientation (Milner *et al.*, 1991). One should therefore be wary of extrapolating from lower-order impairments to assume higher-level problems, as use of multi-modal sensory cues can circumvent early-stage visual difficulties.

Disorders of primary visual processing

At this basic level of visual analysis, separate aspects of the visual world are processed bilaterally. Selective impairments are therefore only likely to arise with large lesions compromising both occipital lobes, but patients have been reported with specific deficits in a range of visual functions including appreciation of color, depth, shape, size, and location (Warrington, 1986), and movement (Zihl *et al.*, 1983). Additionally, loss of ability to differentiate figure from ground can occur as an early visual deficit in the context of preserved visual form discrimination (Kartsounis and Warrington, 1991).

Recent *f*MRI studies have suggested that input from higher-order visual areas (V4 for color, V5 for motion) may mediate recovery in lower-order V1 lesions after stroke, by providing contralesional activation transmitted via the corpus callosum (Raposo *et al.*, 2011). The authors argue that this early cerebral reorganization could be a target for rehabilitation, and propose that visual restoration therapies should be evaluated during the acute phase to capitalize on this plasticity. The window of opportunity in stroke is brief, however, and lack of resources is a major barrier to exploiting this recovery potential. There is clearly scope for technological devices to assist in this regard as they can deliver repeated stimulation in consistent fashion that can be very accurately calibrated and evaluated.

Disorders of visual perception and recognition

Visual form agnosia

The neurologist, Lissauer, is credited with introducing a distinction which is still used today between failure of visual recognition due to impaired perception and that due to damage to stored knowledge about objects (Lissauer, 1890). The term "apperceptive agnosia" refers to the former – any failure of visual recognition attributable to poor perception. The problems may be due to impairments in any of a number of perceptual attributes (visual form agnosia; Benson and Greenberg, 1969) or their integration (Riddoch and Humphreys, 1987), hence this term refers to a heterogeneous range of disorders.

Early attempts at remediation involved practicing visuo-spatial tasks focusing more on psychometric measures rather than real-world benefits (Young *et al.*, 1983; Gordon *et al.*, 1985). Results were generally rather negative (Edmans and Lincoln, 1991). Given the variability of perceptual disorders, current approaches favor a more bespoke analysis of the deficits, although a sophisticated theoretical assessment is often followed by a basic common-sense approach to rehabilitation. Intervention, beyond providing education about the problems, usually involves changing the environment, either by minimizing distracting cues or otherwise to highlight salient perceptual attributes of objects. A third common technique is to use verbal labels to circumvent reliance on visual cues, though reading can also be affected by severe perceptual deficits. Wilson (1999) described a college student with perceptual deficits who benefited from basic strategies such as keeping his mug in a different place from his peers, and having written labels to identify clothes. A number of educational, cueing, and environmental restructuring strategies are suggested by Shaw (2001).

Prosopagnosia

Prosopagnosia is a specific disorder in identifying familiar faces and is particularly disabling from a psychological perspective. Prosopagnosia is most often associated with left posterior lesions (Meadows, 1974), the cause being a higher-order dysfunction in either face recognition or stored representations of personal identity (Humphreys and Bruce, 1989), though McNeil and Warrington (1991) suggested that the distinction is between damage to face recognition units and their disconnection, the latter being capable of covert facial recognition.

There are few rehabilitation studies for this fascinating condition. DeGutis *et al.* (2007) treated congenital prosopagnosia with tasks involving learning to discriminate faces by spatial configuration. Training was linked to increased functional connectivity in ventral temporal-occipital face selective regions on *f*MRI. This is a single case and more evidence is clearly needed as to the utility of this method. Unfortunately, training tends to be extensive and time-consuming, well beyond the remit of a normal clinical service, and not always successful (e.g. Wilson, 1987; De Haan *et al.*, 1991). Ellis and Young's (1988) child prosopagnosic spent a full school year receiving daily treatment in over 1,000 sessions with little impact on face identification. However, as these kinds of task are easily automated, it should be possible to develop packages which can be delivered efficiently and thereby contribute to larger-scale studies of treatment effectiveness.

Simultanagnosia

Simultanagnosia is a condition characterized by the inability to integrate multiple objects into a coherent whole. The individual objects are perceived, but patients have difficulty describing a complex scene and the overall meaning is lost. Coslett and Saffran (1990) suggested that it results from a disconnection between structural descriptions of objects (the "what" system) and coding of object location (the "where"). The size of the objects is irrelevant; it is the number of objects that causes the problem. Thus, reading is often difficult. One of the first author's patients with a mild form of this condition reported that he had difficulty seeing more than two objects on a table or discriminating two objects if they were overlapping.

Farah (1990) distinguishes between dorsal and ventral simultanagnosia, the latter retaining the ability to see multiple objects but not to recognize them.

Simultanagnosia is one cardinal feature of Balint's Syndrome, which is also characterized by defective visually-guided hand movements (optic ataxia) and inability to direct the eyes toward a target (ocular apraxia). Although this triad of symptoms has been much debated (Rizzo, 1993), their frequent co-occurrence reminds us that perceptual disorders are complex and rarely occur in isolation. Roselli et al. (2001) reported a rehabilitation single case study of Balint's Syndrome with good functional outcome using a range of strategies that included practicing real-life tasks. Zgaljardic et al. (2011) reported some success with a multi-modal intervention for six hours a day, five days a week, which included a range of visual exercises. Again, however, the intervention is intensive and could be compromised by fatigue or poor motivation.

This is a challenging but intriguing condition which has not been considered suitable for assistive technology to date. Yet, visual attention deficits are a common contributor to poor visual perception. In both the design of specific training exercises, and in development of everyday household systems, there is considerable potential for new technologies to be recruited to improve function and perhaps reduce impairment.

Visual neglect

Perhaps the most widely recognized disorder of visual attention is visual neglect, characterized as inattention to one aspect of the visual array. This complex condition takes various forms; for example, although it is usually a deficit of lateralized attention (i.e. to the right or left side) it may occur vertically (altitudinal neglect; Butter et al., 1989). Neglect is most common after right hemisphere lesions and therefore usually affects the left portions of stimuli. Studies of stroke patients with neglect have implicated the medical temporal parahippocampal region and angular gyrus of the inferior parietal lobe gyrus (Mort et al., 2003) as well as the frontal lobes (Husain and Kennard, 1996), but presentations vary considerably. Spatial neglect is characterized by omission of stimuli to one side of space, whereas object-centered neglect involves inattention to portions of each object in an array regardless of position.

Many different treatments have been tried for neglect, including eye-patching, vibration, caloric stimulation, and auditory feedback (see the excellent review by Robertson and Halligan, 1999). Commonly, a visual cue is presented in the neglected space to re-orient attention to that side, although cues presented in the non-neglected side may be more effective by re-orienting a right hemisphere global attention system (Halligan and Marshall, 1994). More active cueing strategies involving recruitment of limbs contralateral to the lesion can reduce neglect (Halligan and Marshall, 1989; Robertson and North, 1993; Worthington, 1996) though the left limb advantage in reducing unilateral left neglect is reduced when activated in right hemispace (Halligan et al., 1991), suggesting that the spatio-motor cueing aspect of this technique is crucial rather than hemispheric activation per se. Humphreys and Riddoch (1994b) and Riddoch et al. (1995) proposed that cueing modality interacts with the neglect subtype so that visual cues may be more effective with deficits in orienting visual attention, and motor strategies are optimal for deficits initiating actions within spatial reference frames (see also Riddoch et al., 1995). Early attempts to use computer technology were disappointing (Robertson et al., 1990), but new technologies, such as virtual reality, may prove more useful in providing realistic training scenarios for this debilitating condition (Tsirlin et al., 2009; see also Chapter 2, this volume).

Associative agnosia

The associative agnosias are characterized by an inability to associate knowledge about an object from its form. Perception is intact but, in Hans Teuber's famous phrase, is stripped of its meaning. This may arise from a problem linking perceptual information about an object to knowledge about its function; for example, not recognizing a handle on a cup as the means to grasp it, or from inability to access stored knowledge about an object's function. This can also lead to deficits in recognizing faces (Prosopagnosia) or recognizing words or letters (Pure alexia). In daily life, these deficits can cause considerable problems as people may be unable to use tools and relate to common objects necessary for everyday living.

Therapies for agnosia have been attempted with limited success, though re-learning old knowledge may be easier than trying to acquire new information (Swales and Johnson, 1992). Helping patients to access old knowledge may therefore be a useful treatment technique for many, but perhaps not all. Even when effective, treatment gains may not generalize. Francis et al. (2001) used mnemonics to help an agnosic man re-learn his letters. Therapy was extensive (the letter X took 10 weeks to recognize), and there was some generalization to whole read reading (80 percent accuracy), although additional therapy was required to train him to read irregular words and this did not result in a return to normal reading. A similar cautionary note was sounded by Francis et al. (2002) in treating a prosopagnosic woman: despite statistically significant improvements using a highly contrived compensatory strategy, she continued to have difficulty recognizing people in daily life. Similarly Wilson (1999) taught an agnosic woman to identify objects (correctly naming 89/93 objects on which she was trained), but this seemed to work more by a process of specific pairing of verbal label and visual pattern; the results did not generalize to daily life (only naming 6/52 control stimuli).

This is an area where there is great scope for new technological innovation, perhaps by automatizing intensive training practice (though evidence is slim for its effectiveness), but, more promisingly, by developing computer vision systems to compensate for impaired visual recognition, for example by providing audio cues to inform a user of an object's identity or its function. Systems might also give auditory description of features of objects such that the user can use the correct item in sequence, such as making coffee. There are considerable opportunities for clinicians, developers, and engineers to work collaboratively on these kinds of projects with the potential to transform the lives of those afflicted by visual perceptual impairment.

Current and emerging visual technologies

Recently, the applications of computer vision to extend visual accessibility have been blossoming. While most approaches tend to focus on very narrow sub-problems, and generally aim at the visually impaired and blind community, they suggest many possibilities for study and potential application in the specific areas outlined above. The rapid progress of technology – computational power, optical clarity, energy efficiency, and portability of devices, coupled with dramatic progress in computer vision algorithms, are a powerful tool to help understand and augment human activities.

A number of different approaches have been taken to the problem of visual object recognition, which is key to any assistive technology for the visually- or perceptually-impaired. Bigham *et al.* (2010) developed an app that facilitates answering of visually-based questions through Mechanical Turk (human-powered recognition) solutions (Amazon, 2013). The iOS app called VizWiz allows a person to take an image and record a question about it to be answered by the social network. The preferences allow control over the choice of social networks to deploy the question. They include email, web workers, image recognition engine IQEngines (IQEngines, 2013), Twitter, or Facebook. The app is simple to use and delivers satisfactory results. Since the web workers are participating in an online marketplace for their services, VizWiz has created a complex structure of incentives to motivate them to answer questions in a timely fashion. With the managed incentives, the answer arrives in under a minute. Users need to be able to tolerate this delay, but for certain activities it could prove helpful in overcoming an obstacle to task completion, such as preparing a meal or reading a specific word. If the item in question was not properly framed in the photo, another query must be sent.

In January 2013 TapTapSee was launched (TapTapSee, 2013). This object identification app features a minimal human interface with just three buttons and a preview of the video. A double-tap initiates an image recognition query to a large network of humans prepared to manually describe the image contents in a couple of descriptive words (Tag Pics, 2013). The simpler interface makes the application easier to use and accessible to a broader population. As the answers come from people, not machines, most image queries can be successfully described. Automated systems are limited by the explicit content within the available databases. Apps of this kind have great potential to provide real-time information for people with disorders of form perception and recognition. In cases where functional knowledge has been lost, naming or describing an object may not assist a person to use it correctly.

For more than 40 years, persons who are blind have stated consistently that any device that makes them appear strange, unusual, or otherwise attracts undue attention, is a non-starter (Pullin, 2009). This was an issue with the Sonic Guide (Brabyn, 1982) of the mid-1970s. The desirability of consumer electronics and smartphones such as the iPhone is an advantage in this respect. Apple iOS devices are available off-the-shelf and popular among visually impaired and sighted users. They unify a variety of accessibility, daily living, and communication needs, all in one unit. As a platform, they are open to developers to make custom applications that make use of their camera, sensors, and computational power. It is easy to connect other peripherals and sensors to them via Bluetooth or via the headphone jack, allowing for a wide range of physical and spatial interfaces.

Coughlan and Manduchi (2009) present an automated mobile wayfinding system based on strategically placed colored markers. This has potential for those with topographical disorientation due to inability to recognize familiar surroundings. The system works within a controlled environment and could in principle be customized to a user's immediate locality. Their recent studies (Manduchi and Coughlan, 2014) suggest that appropriate feedback from camera-based technologies helps train accurate proprioceptive responses. With a different approach, Košecká et al. (2005) successfully demonstrated the feasibility of using scale-invariant feature transform descriptors (Lowe, 2004) for global localization and relative pose estimation. Keypoint descriptors invariant to scale and orientation can be used to build a 3D map of the environment and subsequently used to determine one's position by location recognition. While their work is developed within the context of robotics and a comparably dense dataset, their results have direct impact in our application. In a related extension, Hile et al. (2009) combined GPS information and image-based reconstruction to create a model of the desired environment, to then compute a navigational path for a pedestrian.

Several teams (Merler et al., 2007; Winlock et al., 2010) have been working on a shopping assistant for the visually impaired. Their multi-faceted approach reveals some of the complexities and depth of the problem. In designing the hardware from scratch, they gain the ability for more refined haptic feedback to aid with localization of the items. In time, this kind of approach could prove beneficial for a range of visual disorders including visual neglect, loss of object recognition, and simultanagnosia.

Chen and Yuille (2004) have proposed a framework for real-time text detection and reading text in city scenes. Their work aims to serve text-based information to a visually impaired person while navigating an urban environment. Their approach assumes that the person can anticipate a text region of interest in the environment and is capable of aiming a still camera at it to send to a server for processing. The results are very impressive; however, text-only processing and reliance solely on still images limit the system. In July 2012, Blindsight released the Text Detective app (Text Detective, 2013) featuring the text detection and recognition algorithms based on the work of Chen and Yuille. This has promise, but, like a lot of these technologies, the quality of the photograph can affect the usefulness of the system, and taking an adequate photograph may be more difficult for some visually impaired than others.

Google Goggles is an image-based search engine from Google (Google, 2013). The engine performs text detection and recognition combined with image-based recognition to determine the content of the image. Google provides the Goggles functionality in their Google app on iOS. This capability will hopefully soon be accessible to the visually impaired via the VoiceOver interface.

The reality of computer vision applications for the visually impaired has not yet seen significant adoption, with most people relying on low-tech but very reliable "technologies" such as the cane, guide dogs, folding bills, and using rubber bands and safety pins to identify objects. While there are mobile optical character recognition readers on the market (Kurzweil/National Federation for the Blind (KNFB) Reading Technology, 2013), their cost and limitations make them currently inaccessible. Dedicated laser barcode readers can identify various items, but are bulky, expensive, and address only the items with barcodes. To address these limitations, we combined some of the best implementations of computer vision available today, and now present an affordable, accessible, and comprehensive platform for computer-aided visual assistance that runs on a wide range of off-the-shelf smartphones.

At this time, currency in the United States is not accessible to blind or visually impaired persons. In many other countries, the bill designs include a variety of features such as different sizes for each denomination, very different colors, and large numbers to help those with low-vision and, in some cases, even Braille markings. Absence of these elements in the design of United States currency typically necessitates the use of specialized hardware assistive technologies such as the iBill or the Franklin Bill Reader Money Identifier. These are dedicated hardware devices designed solely to identify US currency. They are powered by AAA batteries and are approximately 3" × 2" × 1" in size. They combine a small camera, an embedded processor, and custom software for currency identification. Given the general-purpose computational capabilities of smartphones, coupled with iOS's VoiceOver accessibility foundation, LookTel sought to address money identification by deploying the image recognition engine directly on the iPhone, and related iOS devices. The iOS platform with an accessible method for distributing the app through the Apple App Store created an unparalleled method to distribute the technology at an affordable cost. The app, LookTel Money Reader, is simple. Like its physical analogs, it is designed to only do one thing: recognize bills easily and reliably. Once the app is started, the iOS device itself becomes the human interface. One points the camera at the bills to be identified, and listens to the denominations as they are read by VoiceOver. There is a minimal human interface. When used without VoiceOver, the app plays pre-synthesized audio descriptions of all bills. When used with VoiceOver, the app synthesizes each description on the fly. A tap on the screen while nothing is actively being recognized triggers an announcement of Money Reader's readiness. This provides feedback that the system is functioning correctly. This feedback proves invaluable for persons initially learning how to best aim the camera as it gives guidance that the bill in question is not in view of the camera. The speed of Money Reader, 20 frames per second on the iPhone 4, and 30 frames per second on the iPhone 5, combined with the accuracy of the recognition system, is good enough to enhance a person's ability to coordinate quickly through proprioception the relative bill to camera positions.

Many people start by placing the phone flat on the bill and then slowly pulling the phone away. After several successful recognitions, people learn the optimal range for moving the bill into the field of view of the phone's camera. LookTel often receives direct feedback from people who use the Money Reader app. Though still in usability rather than rehabilitative trials, most comments are very positive. Users have expressed appreciation for the app's ease of use. Instructors and rehabilitation specialists find the app reliable and intuitive and have been recommending its use. The real-time feedback, with recognition, affords rapid proprioceptive learning. The extension of the hands now offers a fast-enough feedback for muscle memory to learn relative position of both hands while keeping the bill within the view of the camera. The simplicity of use and rapid feedback are very important for people new to the concept of a camera. We have heard from several individuals who have started working as cashiers, using the Money Reader as a tool.

Since the initial release of the LookTel Money Reader in 2011, the subsequent updates have added 19 additional currencies, all supported simultaneously – Australian Dollar, Bahraini Dinar, Brazilian Real, Belarusian Ruble, British Pound, Canadian Dollar, Euro, Hungarian Forint, Israeli Shekel, Indian Rupee, Japanese Yen, Kuwaiti Dinar, Mexican Peso, New Zealand Dollar, Polish Zloty, Russian Ruble, Saudi Arabian Riyal, Singapore Dollar, and United Arab Emirates Dirham.

After the success of the Money Reader, LookTel redesigned the core recognition element within the context of iOS to deliver a mechanism for real-time object recognition. The LookTel Recognizer app was designed for blind and visually impaired persons who can benefit from a technology to assist in identifying objects. Recognizer permits people to store images of objects in a database, and then have the iOS device quickly recognize these items when scanned with the camera. This is an open-ended system that allows instant object recognition.

The Recognizer app utilizes real-time recognition capabilities with customization that permits a flexible range of ways to use it – identifying everyday objects such as packaged goods, identity cards, canned foods, or CDs in a music collection. Following the approach used in Money Reader, LookTel minimized the human interface. The app is built around capturing items for the database, and recognizing them later. On the main screen, the recognition sequence is always running, and will announce a known item anytime it is in the field of view. A double-tap on the main preview screen captures the image for the database, termed a library, and initiates the recording of the audio label.

The database of trained items is stored locally on the device allowing the editing, adding, removing, and relabeling of individual items. The database can be emailed for sharing or backup purposes, as can individual items. Entirely local processing of the image recognition and training removes unnecessary delays and complications. The customer no longer has to manage a backend engine on another computer, nor do they need to rely on any network connectivity. Decoupling these layers from the task of item recognition, the Recognizer allows customers to backup and export databases via email. This enables them to restore a database from lost or replaced devices, or share it with other members of the community. A barcode scanner is included to provide alternative identification and supplemental information helpful for labeling.

A system like the Recognizer app may have applications for various rehabilitative applications. For example, training all the relevant items in a person's home may assist with agnosia rehabilitation as it could provide support and reinforcement whenever needed. For prosopagnosia, all the family and friends photographs could be entered into the app for instant recall and vocal description of the individuals in those photos – whether they are individual photos, in an album or framed on a wall.

Computer vision and related technologies are opening up many possibilities for supporting rehabilitation and activities of daily living. With image and object recognition capabilities, real-time feedback enables repeated reinforcement agnosia training throughout the day and not just limited to sessions with a specialist. Image recognition with photographs, or more specialized facial recognition algorithms, can support interactive exercises aimed at prosopagnosia rehabilitation. Technologies such as depth-sensing cameras (whether using time-of-flight or structured light technologies) allow for accurate 3D position tracking, pose estimation, activity, and gesture recognition. These systems permit increasingly complex assessments, for example for visual neglect, by tracking the progress of a meal and reminding that a portion of it remained untouched, or to aid with dressing: to ensure the completeness or consistency of one's outfit. With accurate pose and gesture tracking, one can track vestibular balance and fluidity of movement over time, highlighting specific tasks that need most improvement.

Conclusion

Visual perceptual disorders are complex and challenging to clinicians. With a small evidence-base to work from it is perhaps unsurprising that some contemporary textbooks on cognitive rehabilitation omit visual rehabilitation completely (Sohlberg and Mateer, 2001; Ponsford, 2004; Halligan and Wade, 2005). Likewise, in their literature review, Gillespie *et al.* (2012) found no clinical trials of assistive technology for perceptual disorders. Yet, as Anderson (2002) acknowledged, "it would seem that many of the critical elements are in place for major advances in the neuropsychological rehabilitation of visuoperceptual disorders" (2002: 179). Inability to interact with the world visually threatens our independence and capacity for social participation. The technologies we have reviewed here have the potential to provide new possibilities for therapy and compensation for these most debilitating of cognitive disorders.

References

Amazon (2013). Available at: www.mturk.com/ (accessed 26 September 2014).

Anderson, S. W. (2002). Visuoperceptual Impairments. In Eslinger, P. J. (ed.), *Neuropsychological Interventions* (pp. 163–181). New York, NY: The Guilford Press.

Balliet, R., Blood, R. M. T., and Bacy-Y-Rita, P. (1985). Visual Field Rehabilitation in the Cortically Blind? *Journal of Neurology, Neurosurgery and Psychiatry*, 48: 1113–24.

Benson, D. F. and Greenberg, J. P. (1969). Visual Form Agnosia. *Archives of Neurology*, 20: 82–9.

Bigham, J. P., Jayant, C., Ji, H., Little, G., Miller, R., Miller, R. C., Tatrowicz, A., White, B., White, S., and Yeh, T. (2010). VizWiz: Nearly Real-Time Answers to Visual Questions. In *Proceedings of the 23rd Annual ACM Symposium on User Interface Software and Technology* (pp. 333–42). New York, NY: ACM.

Bouwmeester, L., Heutink, J., and Cees, L. (2007). The Effects of Visual Training for Patients with Visual Field Defects due to Brain Damage: A Systematic Review. *Journal of Neurology, Neurosurgery and Psychiatry*, 78: 555–64.

Brabyn, J. A. (1982). New Developments in Mobility and Orientation Aids for the Blind. *IEEE Transactions on Biomedical Engineering*, 29(4): 285–9.

Butter, C. M., Evans, J., Kirsch, N., and Kewman, D. (1989). Altitudinal Neglect Following Traumatic Brain Injury: A Case Report. *Cortex*, 25: 135–46.

Chen, X. and Yuille, A. L. (2004). Detecting and Reading Text in Natural Scenes. In *Proceedings of the 2004 IEEE Conference on Computer Vision and Pattern Recognition* (Vol. 2, pp. II–366), Washington, DC, USA.

Coslett, H. B. and Saffran, E. (1990). Simultanagnosia: To See But Not Two See. *Brain*, 114(4): 1523–45.

Coughlan, J. and Manduchi, R. (2009). Functional Assessment of a Camera Phone-Based Wayfinding System Operated by Blind and Visually Impaired Users. *International Journal on Artificial Intelligence Tools*, 18(3): 379–97.

DeGutis, J. M., Shlomo, B., Robertson, L. C., and D'Esposito, M. (2007). Functional Plasticity in Ventral Temporal Cortex Following Cognitive Rehabilitation of a Congenital Prosopagnosic. *Journal of Cognitive Neuroscience*, 19(11): 1790–802.

De Haan, E. H. F., Young, A. W., and Newcombe, F. (1991). Covert and Overt Recognition in Prosopagnosia. *Brain*, 114: 2757–91.

Edmans, J. A. and Lincoln, N. B. (1991). Treatment of Visual Perceptual Deficits after Stroke: Single Case Studies on Four Patients with Right Hemiplegia. *British Journal of Occupational Therapy*, 54: 139–44.

Ellis, A. and Young, A. (1988). Training in Face-Processing Skills for a Child with Acquired Prosopagnosia. *Developmental Neuropsychology*, 4: 283–94.

Farah, M. J. (1990). *Visual Agnosia*. Cambridge, MA: MIT Press.

Francis, D. R., Riddoch, M. J., and Humphreys, G. W. (2001). Treating Agnosic Alexia Complicated by Additional Impairments. *Neuropsychological Rehabilitation*, 11(2): 113–92.

Francis, D. R., Riddoch, M. J., and Humphreys, G. W. (2002). 'Who's That Girl?' Prosopagnosia, Person-Based Semantic Disorder, and the Reacquisition of Face Identification. *Neuropsychological Rehabilitation*, 12(1): 1–26.

Friedman, P. J. and Leong, L. (1992). Perceptual Impairment After Stroke: Improvements During the First Three Months. *Disability and Rehabilitation*, 14(3): 136–9.

Gillespie, A., Best, C., and O'Neill, B. (2012). Cognitive Function and Assistive Technology for Cognition: A Systematic Review. *Journal of the International Neuropsychological Society*, 18: 1–19.

Google (2013). Available at: www.google.com/mobile/goggles/ (accessed 26 September 2014).

Gordon, W. A., Hibbard, M. R., Egeiko, S., Diller, L., Shaver, M. S., Lieberman, A., and Ragnarsson, K. (1985). Perceptual Remediation in Patients with Right Brain Damage: A Comprehensive Program. *Archives of Physical Medicine and Rehabilitation*, 66: 353–59.

Halligan, P. W. and Marshall, J. C. (1989). Laterality of Motor Response in Visuo-Spatial Neglect: A Case Study. *Neuropsychologia*, 27: 1301–07.

Halligan, P. W. and Marshall, J. C. (1994). Focal and Global: Attention Modulates the Expression of Visuo-Spatial Neglect: A Case Study. *Neuropsychologia*, 32(1): 13–21.

Halligan, P. W. and Wade, D. T. (2005). *Effectiveness of Rehabilitation for Cognitive Deficits*. New York, NY: Oxford University Press.

Halligan, P. W., Manning, L., and Marshall, J. C. (1991). Hemispheric Activation Vs Spatio-Motor Cueing in Visual Neglect: A Case Study. *Neuropsychologia*, 29: 165–76.

Hile, H., Grzeszczuk, R., Liu, A., Vedantham, R., Košecká, J., and Borriello, G. (2009). Landmark-based Pedestrian Navigation with Enhanced Spatial Reasoning. In *Pervasive Computing* (pp. 59–76). New York, NY: Springer.

Humphreys, G. W. and Bruce, V. (1989). *Visual Cognition: Computational, Experimental and Neuropsychological Perspectives*. Hove, UK: Lawrence Erlbaum Associates.

Humphreys, G. W. and Riddoch, M. J. (1994a). Visual Object Processing in Normality and Pathology: Implications for Rehabilitation. In Riddoch, M.J. and Humphreys, G.W. (eds), *Cognitive Neuropsychology and Cognitive Rehabilitation* (pp. 39–76). Hove, UK: Lawrence Erlbaum Associates.

Humphreys, G. W. and Riddoch, M. J. (1994b). Attention to Within-Object and Between-Object Spatial Representations: Multiple Sites for Visual Selection. *Cognitive Neuropsychology*, 11: 207–41.

Husain, M. and Kennard, C. (1996). Visual Neglect Associated with Frontal Lobe Infarction. *Journal of Neurology*, 243: 652–57.

IQEngines (2013). Available at: www.iqengines.com (accessed 26 September 2014).

Jackowski, M. M., Sturr, J. F., Taub, H. A., and Turk, M. A. (1996). Photophobia in Patients with Traumatic Brain Injury: Use of Light-Filtering Lenses to Enhance Contrast Sensitivity and Reading Rate. *NeuroRehabilitation*, 6: 193–201.

Kartsounis, L. D. and Warrington, E. K. (1991). Failure of Object Recognition due to a Breakdown of Figure-Ground Discrimination in a Patient with Normal Acuity. *Neuropsychologia*, 29(10): 969–80.

Košecká, J., Li, F., and Yang, X. (2005). Global Localization and Relative Positioning based on Scale-Invariant Keypoints. *Robotics and Autonomous Systems*, 52(1): 27–38.

Kurzweil/National Federation for the Blind (KNFB) Reading Technology (2013). Available at: www.knfbreader.com/ (accessed 26 September 2014).

Lissauer, H. (1890). Ein fall von Seelenblindheit Nebst Einem Beitrage zur Theorie Derselben. *Archiv fur Psychiatrie und Nervenkrankheiten*, 21: 222–70.

Lowe, D. G. (2004). Distinctive Image Features from Scale-Invariant Keypoints. *International Journal of Computer Vision*, 60(2): 91–110.

McNeil, J. and Warrington, E. K. (1991). Prosopagnosia: A Reclassification. *The Quarterly Journal of Experimental Psychology*, 43A(2): 267–87.

Manduchi, R. and Coughlan, J. (2014). The Last Meter: Blind Visual Guidance to a Target. In *Proceedings of the SIGCHI Conference on Human Factors in Computing Systems*. Available at: www.escholarship.org/uc/item/7hc5p9p1 (accessed 26 September 2014).

Marr, D. (1982). *Vision*. San Francisco, CA: W. H. Freeman.

Meadows, J. C. (1974). The Anatomical Basis of Prosopagnosia. *Journal of Neurology, Neurosurgery and Psychiatry*, 37: 489–501.

Merler, M., Galleguillos, C., and Belongie, S. (2007). Recognizing Groceries in situ Using In-Vitro Training Data. In *IEEE Conference on Computer Vision and Pattern Recognition 2007* (pp. 1–8), Minneapolis, MN, USA.

Milner, A. D. and Goodale, M. A. (1995). *The Visual Brain in Action*. Oxford, UK: Oxford University Press.

Milner, A. D., Perrett, D. I., Johnston, R. S., Benson, P. J., Jordan, T. R., Heeley, D. W., Bettucci, D., Mortara, F., Mutani, R., Terazzi, E., and Davidson, D. L. W. (1991). Perception and Action in Visual Form Agnosia. *Brain*, 114: 405–28.

Mort, D. J., Malhotra, P., Mannan, S. K., Rorden, C., Parnbakian, A., Kennard, C., and Husain, M. (2003). The Anatomy of Visual Neglect. *Brain*, 126(9): 1986–97.

Politzer, T. A. (1996). Case Studies of a New Approach Using Partial and Selective Occlusion for the Clinical Treatment of Diplopia. *NeuroRehabilitation*, 6: 213–17.

Ponsford, J. (2004). *Cognitive and Behavioral Rehabilitation*. New York, NY: The Guilford Press.

Poppelreuter, W. (1917/1990). *Disturbances of Lower and Higher Visual Capacities Caused by Occipital Damage*. Oxford, UK: Clarendon Press.

Pullin, G. (2009). *Design Meets Disability*. Cambridge, MA: MIT Press.

Raposo, N., Cauquil, A. S., Acket, B., Celebrini, S., Pariente, J., Cognard, C., Loubinoux, I., and Chollet, F. (2011). Post Stroke Conscious Visual Deficit: Clinical Course and Changes in Cerebral Activations. *Neurorehabilitation and Neural Repair*, 25(8): 703–10.

Resnikoff, S., Pascolini, D., Etya'ale, D., Kocur, I., Pararajasegaram, R., Pokahrel, G. P., and Mariotti, S. P. (2004). Global Data on Visual Impairment in the Year 2002. *Bulletin of the World Health Organization*, 82: 844–51.

Riddoch, M. J. and Humphreys, G. W. (1987). A Case of Integrative Visual Agnosia. *Brain*, 110: 1431–62.

Riddoch, M. J., Humphreys, G. W., Burroughs, E., Luckhurst, L., Bateman, A., and Hill, S. (1995). Cueing in a Case of Neglect: Modality an Automaticity Effects. *Cognitive Neuropsychology*, 12: 605–21.

Rizzo, M. (1993). "Balint's Syndrome" and Associated Visuospatial Disorders. In Kennard, C. (ed.), *Balliere's Clinical Neurology: Visual Perceptual Defects* (pp. 415–37). London, UK: Balliere Tindall.

Robertson, I. H. and North, N. T. (1993). Active and Passive Activation of Left Limbs: Influence on Sensory Neglect. *Neuropsychologia*, 31: 293–300.

Robertson, I. H. and Halligan, P. W. (1999). *Spatial Neglect: A Clinical Handbook for Diagnosis and Treatment*. Hove, UK: Psychology Press.

Robertson, I. H., Gray, J. M., Pentland, B., and Waite, L. J. (1990). Microcomputer-based Rehabilitation for Unilateral Left Visual Neglect: A Randomized Controlled Trial. *Archives of Physical Medicine and Rehabilitation*, 71: 663–68.

Roselli, M., Ardila, A., and Beltran, C. (2001). Rehabilitation of Balint's Syndrome: A Single Case Report. *Applied Neuropsychology*, 8: 242–47.

Rossi, P. W., Kheyfets, S., and Reding, M. J. (1990). Fresnel Prisms Improve Visual Perception in Stroke Patients with Homonymous Hemianopia or Unilateral Visual Neglect. *Neurology*, 40(10): 1597.

Rowe, F., Brand, D., Jackson, C. A., Price, A., Walker, L., Harrison, S., Eccleston, C., Scott, C., Akerman, N., Dodridge, C., Howard, C., Shipman, T., Sperring, U., MacDiarmid, S., and Freeman, C. (2009). Visual impairment Following Stroke: Do Stroke Patients Require Vision Assessment? *Age and Ageing*, 38: 188–93.

Schuett, S., Heywood, C. A., Kentridge, R. W., Dauner, R., and Zihl, J. (2012). Rehabilitation of Reading and Visual Field Disorders: Transfer or Specificity? *Brain*, 135(3): 912–21.

Shaw, J. (2001). The Assessment and Rehabilitation of Visuo-Spatial Disorders. In Johnstone, B. and Stonnington, H. H. (eds), *Rehabilitation of Neuropsychological Disorders* (pp. 125–60). Hove, UK: Psychology Press.

Sohlberg, M. M. and Mateer, C. A. (2001). *Cognitive Rehabilitation. An Integrative Neuro-psychological Approach*. New York, NY: The Guilford Press.

Swales, M. and Johnson, R. (1992). Patients with Sematic Memory Loss: Can They Relearn Lost Concepts? *Neuropsychological Rehabilitation*, 2(4): 295–305.

Tag Pics. Image Searcher, Inc. (2013). Available at: www.tagpics.net (accessed 26 September 2014).

TapTapSee (2013). Available at: www.taptapseeapp.com/ (accessed 26 September 2014).

Text Detective, Blindsight LLC. (2013). Available at: http://blindsight.com/textdetective/ (accessed 26 September 2014).

Tsirlin, I., Dupierrix, E., Chokron, S., Coquillart, S., and Ohlmann, T. (2009). Uses of Virtual Reality for Diagnosis, Rehabilitation and Study of Unilateral Spatial Neglect: Review and Analysis. *CyberPsychology and Behavior*, 12(2): 175–81.

Ungerleider, L. G. and Mishkin, M. (1982). Two Cortical Visual Systems. In Ingle, J., Goodale, M. A., and Mansfield, R. J. W. (eds), *Analysis of Visual Behaviour* (pp. 549–86). Cambridge, MA: MIT Press.

Vitale, S., Cotch, M. F., and Spreduto, R. D. (2006). Prevalence of Visual Impairment in the United States. *Journal of the American Medical Association*, 295(18): 2158–63.

Warren, M. (1993). A Hierarchical Model for Evaluation and Treatment of Visual Perceptual Dysfunction in Adult Acquired Brain Injury. *American Journal of Occupational Therapy*, 47: 42–66.

Warrington, E. K. (1986). Visual Deficits Associated with Occipital Lobe Lesions in Man. *Experimental Brain Research Supplementum, Series II* (pp 247–61). Berlin, Germany: Springer-Verlag.

Wilson, B. (1987). *Rehabilitation of Memory*. London, UK: Guilford Press.

Wilson, B. A. (1999). *Case Studies in Neuropsychological Rehabilitation*. New York, NY: Oxford University Press.

Winlock, T., Christiansen, E., and Belongie, S. (2010). Toward Real-Time Grocery Detection for the Visually Impaired. In *IEEE Conference on Computer Vision and Pattern Recognition Workshop 2010* (pp. 49–56), San Francisco, California, USA.

World Health Organisation (2012). *Global Data on Visual Impairments 2010*. Geneva: WHO.

Worthington, A. D. (1996). Cueing Strategies in Neglect Dyslexia. *Neuropsychological Rehabilitation*, 6(1): 1–17.

Worthington, A. D. and Riddoch, M. J. (2008). Visual-Perceptual And Spatio-Motor Disorders. In Tyerman, A. D. and King, N. (eds), *Psychological Approaches to Rehabilitation after Traumatic Brain Injury* (pp. 166–92). Oxford, UK: BPS Blackwell.

Young, G. C., Collins, D., and Hren, M. (1983). Effect of Pairing Scanning Training with Block Design Training in the Remediation of Perceptual Problems in Left Hemiplegics. *Journal of Clinical Neuropsychology*, 5(3): 201–12.

Zgaljardic, D. J., Yancy, S., Levinson, J., Morales, G., and Masel, B. E. (2011). Balint's Syndrome and Post-Acute Brain Injury Rehabilitation: A Case Report. *Brain Injury*, 25(9): 909–17.

Zihl, J. (2011). *Rehabilitation of Visual Disorders after Brain Injury*. Hove, UK: Psychology Press.

Zihl, J. and von Cramon, D. (1979). Restitution of Visual Function in Patients with Cerebral Blindness. *Journal of Neurology, Neurosurgery and Psychiatry*, 42: 312–22.

Zihl, J., von Cramon, D., and Mai, N. (1983). Selective Disturbance of Movement Vision after Bilateral Brain Damage. *Brain*, 106(2): 313–40.

6

ASSISTIVE TECHNOLOGY FOR EXECUTIVE FUNCTIONS

Matthew Jamieson and Jonathan J. Evans

Assistive technology is already in widespread use for physical impairment in the form of wheelchairs, hearing aids, prosthetic limbs, and many others. Although use of assistive technology for cognitive impairments is far less widespread, we will argue here that there is evidence that some aspects of executive functioning may be supported by currently available technologies, and emerging technologies provide scope for creative new ways of improving everyday functioning in people with executive dysfunction.

Executive functioning is the term used to encompass a range of cognitive skills including problem solving, planning, initiation, self-monitoring, and error correction. Executive functions enable us to manage problems that arise in everyday life and to deal with novel situations. They are the cognitive skills we use to identify goals, and work toward them, modifying actions when required (Burgess *et al.*, 2005). Much of everyday life is routine – patterns of action become automatic through repetition. Elements of complex tasks, such as driving, preparing meals, and operating a computer, can be carried out with little conscious attention. However, when a potentially dangerous situation arises, or a novel problem is encountered, attention can be focused on the process of working out how to respond, formulating a plan of action, implementing the plan, monitoring progress, and modifying the plan if necessary.

Executive functions have been inextricably linked to the operations of the frontal lobes, from accounts of the changes in personality experienced by Phineas Gage through to contemporary case examples of patients with marked difficulties in everyday planning and organizational skills (Shallice and Burgess, 1991), and models of regional specialization within the frontal lobes (Stuss and Knight, 2013).

There are many models of executive functions (Norman and Shallice, 1986; Baddeley and Wilson, 1988; Miyake *et al.*, 2000), but all are clear that under this broad construct there are a number of more specific processes. These are reflected in test batteries and questionnaires used to assess executive functioning such as the Behavioural Assessment of the Dysexecutive Syndrome (BADS; Wilson *et al.*, 1997), the Delis Kaplan Executive Function System (DKEFS; Delis *et al.*, 2001), and the Behaviour Rating Inventory of Executive Functioning (BRIEF) (Roth *et al.*, 2014). These processes include problem solving in novel circumstances; planning in an optimal manner while abiding by rules; judgment and decision making; task initiation; self-monitoring; adapting mental set; the ability to switch between tasks, emotional control, and inhibition; the ability to sustain attention; and working memory. This is not an exhaustive list of all the executive processes and there is still debate as to how separable these processes are (Miyake and Shah, 1999).

What is clear is that the areas of the brain responsible for executive processing are very commonly damaged after acquired brain injury and stroke, and are vulnerable to impairment in a wide range of progressive neurological conditions. Difficulties with executive functioning are sometimes relatively hidden compared to other forms of cognitive impairment, such as language, perception, or memory impairment, but executive difficulties disrupt the ability to participate effectively in many aspects of daily living.

In their review of assistive technology for cognition, Gillespie *et al.* (2012) used the World Health Organization International Classification of Functioning (ICF) framework to review applications of technology in relation to specific domains of cognitive functioning. The ICF domain most relevant to executive functions is "higher level cognitive functions," which is divided into those that enable abstraction, organization, and planning (including carrying out plans), time management, cognitive flexibility, insight, judgment, and problem solving. Gillespie *et al.* noted that, where forms of technology have been used to support higher level cognitive functions, this has been most common in relation to assisting with time management and organization and planning functions. They found the majority of technologies that were designed to improve organization and planning were "micro-prompting" systems designed to support step-by-step completion of multi-step tasks. All of the technologies that were designed to help with time management could be considered reminding systems, supporting prospective memory (e.g. prompting to interrupt one task in order to carry out another intended action at the right moment). Based on this finding, the first two types of technology to be addressed in this chapter will be devices that prompt or remind people to carry out intended tasks and devices that guide or micro-prompt people to carry out the sub-steps of a task in a specific order.

Reminding technologies for carrying out intended tasks

Executive functions involved in carrying out intentions

In order to be independent in everyday life it is important to be able to form intentions and then carry them out at a later date. This is referred to as prospective memory (e.g. remembering to go to a doctor's appointment, remembering to pass on a telephone message, remembering to take medication). Prospective memory tasks are, of course, dependent on memory (i.e. remembering the content of the intention), but they also require executive abilities. Problems with planning and organization may lead to difficulties in making plans or setting intentions, and problems with keeping track of plans could also lead to scheduling mistakes. A lack of initiation will mean an intended action is not implemented, even if the action itself is remembered. Similarly, a failure of goal maintenance (maintaining an intention such that it is triggered at the right moment) means an intention is not carried out even though the person has not "forgotten" the intention. We have all had experience of suddenly remembering something we should have done.

There is a distinction between time-based prospective memory tasks, where a task needs to be performed at a set time (e.g. leaving the house to travel to an appointment half an hour before it is due to start), and event-based prospective memory tasks, where the task is prompted by an event (e.g. walking past the shops and remembering you need to buy some milk). Time-based prospective memory tasks are challenging for someone who has difficulty initiating actions or switching between activities. However, event-based prospective memory tasks can also be challenging if people have difficulties sustaining their attention or monitoring their activities or the environment (they might not notice the shop or the link with buying milk may not be triggered).

Reminding technologies

"Low-tech" aids, such as diaries, calendars, and wall charts, are often used by people with brain injuries or degenerative disease who have difficulties with time management and carrying out future intentions, and these are commonly recommended by clinical services (Evans et al., 2003). For many people and many tasks, simple low-tech solutions are effective. The advantage of using higher-tech solutions in place of pencil and paper methods is clear in the context of memory difficulties. Somebody may forget to check a written note, even if it were looked at recently, while an electronic aid can prompt a person about an event at a relevant time. This functional advantage of electronic technology is also relevant for people with executive functioning difficulties as a prompt can have the effect of switching attention to a relevant task.

Personal reminding devices

Several portable personal technologies that provide reminders have been shown to be useful for increasing performance of everyday tasks (Jamieson et al., 2014). Many of these can be linked to external servers allowing reminders to be set remotely. Devices which have been investigated include NeuroPage (Wilson et al., 2001), personal digital assistants (PDAs) (Dowds et al., 2011), mobile phones (Stapleton et al., 2007), and voice recorders (Van Den Broek et al., 2000). The majority of these have been tested with people with acquired brain injury; however, there is also some evidence that these devices would be suitable for people with cognitive impairments as a result of degenerative disease (see Jamieson et al., 2014 for review).

The most researched personal reminding device is the NeuroPage (Wilson et al., 2001). The NeuroPage is a pager to which pre-programmed reminders are automatically sent via a service provided by the Oliver Zangwill Centre (www.neuropage.nhs.uk). NeuroPage improves the frequency of performance of intended everyday tasks, such as attending appointments or taking medication, and is traditionally used as a simple reminding device for people whose main problem is a memory disorder (e.g. people who may forget what has to be done as well as forgetting to do it). However, NeuroPage has also been used with patients whose difficulties are more "dysexecutive" in nature. For example, patient RP (Evans et al., 1998; Fish et al., 2008) had severe initiation difficulties following a stroke, which were compounded by attentional problems – she found it difficult to initiate actions, but when she did manage to do so, she was frequently distracted by irrelevant things in her environment. Evans et al. argued that RP seemed to benefit from the arousing effect of the pager (the loud beep and vibration) to get her started on a task, but this arousal effect also seemed to support her goal maintenance as she was less likely to be distracted mid-task when she was prompted by the NeuroPage.

Patient RP is an example of someone who does not forget *what* she has to do, but fails to do tasks, or does them but not at the right time. Reflecting this distinction between memory for task content and goal maintenance, Fish et al. (2007) gave people who had difficulty performing everyday memory tasks a text message that said "STOP," prompting people to Stop; Think; Organize; Proceed (for more detail, see Chapter 2). These text-alerts were combined with a brief version of a cognitive rehabilitation intervention called Goal Management Training (GMT) which aims to train people to set clear intentions for actions, placing them on a "mental blackboard." The text-alerts prompt the user to check the mental blackboard. Fish et al. found that, on days that text-alerts were received, performance of intended actions was better than on days without alerts. While this case illustrates that the type of prompting given by the NeuroPage can be useful for people with executive dysfunction, it was found that people with executive problems are less likely to maintain the behaviors prompted by the pager, if the pager is withdrawn, compared to patients with no executive difficulties (Fish et al., 2008), suggesting that the pager may need to be used on a long-term basis for this group. Furthermore, people with very severe attention and executive difficulties may not be able to understand its purpose, and so for this sub-group it may not be helpful (Emslie et al., 2007).

NeuroPage is wearable and this could be an important feature for reminding technology. Another example of worn technology are Smart-watches, and these have great potential for reminding because they can give a particularly noticeable reminder; and, because watches are in widespread use, they are potentially less stigmatizing to use than pagers or other PDAs. Feeling conspicuous when using assistive technology in public is an issue which has been highlighted as a barrier to the uptake of assistive technology (Baldwin and Powell, 2011). A single case study has provided tentative evidence that the watch reminder could be an effective form of prompting (Van Hulle and Hux, 2006). Smartphones are another piece of hardware for which ubiquity is an advantage, and recent studies have begun investigating their efficacy for prompting. For example, Google Calendar is implemented on a personal computer (to plan tasks) and linked to a smartphone device (to deliver reminders) (McDonald *et al.*, 2011). It was found that people with acquired brain injury (ABI) successfully carried out 81 percent of their intended tasks with the reminder compared with 55 percent with a pencil and paper reminder (McDonald *et al.*, 2011).

In-home/static

In-home reminding technologies have been developed in recent years that can prompt people to perform household tasks and manage their lives in a domestic setting (Chan *et al.*, 2008). These are forms of technology that use home-based static systems (such as a television) and are not designed to be portable. One example of innovative in-home technology is television assisted prompting (TAP), which delivers multi-modal prompts through a television (Lemoncello *et al.*, 2011b). This device has been shown to be useful for prompting people with ABI to stick to an exercise program (Lemoncello *et al.*, 2011b) and to perform everyday activities (Lemoncello *et al.*, 2011a). In another study it was shown that a care facility fitted with several technological innovations, including using a personal computer to organize a schedule, and having alarms and reminder messages on several kitchen devices, was successful in increasing the everyday independence of people with cognitive problems (Boman *et al.*, 2010a).

All of these devices perform the same basic function – they allow programming of reminders from some source (a company providing a service, caregivers, end users, or some combination of these) and then give a prompt at a set time or after a certain event (e.g. after somebody leaves the cooker on; Boman *et al.*, 2010b). Therefore, these devices can be categorized as "reminding" devices which aid "time management" as defined by the ICF (as described in Gillespie *et al.*, 2012). Since this functionality is universal between these devices, the authors of two separate systematic reviews that examined these studies have suggested that the evidence from all these studies can be combined and both reviews conclude there is strong evidence that the use of reminding technology with this functionality is effective for improving performance on everyday tasks which can be affected by memory difficulties, executive impairment, and other cognitive impairments (Gillespie *et al.*, 2012; Jamieson *et al.*, 2014).

Scheduling and intelligent technology

Most of the technologies described so far have involved fixed prompts for specified tasks delivered at pre-specified times. However, in recent years there has been interest in a new wave of intelligent or ambient technologies that can sense the environment and aim to predict the best time to give a reminder, and therefore do more than simply allow a user to set a reminder and then receive a prompt at a set time.

A recently tested PDA reminding device, which is deliverable on a personal computer and smartphone, is the Planning and Executive Assistant Trainer (PEAT) (De Joode et al., 2013; Levinson, 1997). This device not only alerts, but can process information about events which need to be done along with time constraints in order to create an optimal schedule and prompt based on this schedule. A similar idea was Autominder, which was designed to manage everyday plans based on information about when a task should take place and how long it usually lasts for. An algorithm automatically creates the optimal plan when all the relevant information is given and the system prompts accordingly (Pollack et al., 2003). The problem with this type of system is that it requires a great deal of information before it can make scheduling and prompting decisions. Intelligent systems which can automatically sense surroundings and learn patterns of responding from users could allow scheduling and prompting systems to become more usable as the information required could be gained implicitly (from sensing the surroundings) rather than explicitly (through a user or caregiver programming events).

Intelligent devices can use two types of feedback from the environment to plan their scheduling, time of prompting, and type of prompting. Devices which use feedback from various cues in the user's environment, for example sensing when the oven has been switched on or the fridge opened, can be said to use reactive planning. This can be contrasted with devices which use a mixture of environmental cues and feedback from the user (mixed initiative planning; Simpson et al., 2006). Machine learning of people's habits over time can also be used to allow reliable predictions of behavior and lead to more useful prompting. Intelligent systems are currently being developed which use sensors and feedback from the environment and the user in order to prompt at the right time (see Boger and Mihailidis, 2011 and Rashidi and Mihailidis, 2013 for reviews). Examples of this include an intelligent pill reminder system which senses when the user is performing an activity in order to prompt them when they are most likely to be able to attend to the reminder (Hayes et al., 2009), a system which uses sensors to give context specific prompts to elderly people to use the handrail when walking down the stairs (Snoek et al., 2009), and a system which uses partially observable Markov decision processes to predict the user's activity based on a combination of sensors in the environment and, when necessary, prompted feedback from the user (Chu et al., 2012).

Evidence for the efficacy and acceptability of intelligent reminding devices is still being gathered. This area of research is likely to grow as technology advances and as the need to reduce the strain on care and support services increases. There is good evidence that reminding devices can support the performance of everyday tasks which are negatively impacted by executive difficulties, such as failing to switch between tasks and failing to initiate or inhibit behaviors (de Joode et al., 2010), although it is difficult to separate executive dysfunction from memory difficulties in the context of everyday activities. There is growing interest in supplementing the prompting functionality of reminding devices with organization support functionality. This functionality is very promising if it can be coupled with advancing intelligent technology innovations which can sense and gain feedback from the user and their surroundings.

Micro-prompting technologies for organization and planning

Executive functions involved in everyday tasks with sub-steps

Independent living involves many multi-step tasks. They range from personal tasks such as completing a morning routine, cooking breakfast, and completing household chores, such as laundry, to leisure and social activities, and performing tasks during paid work. In all these areas, there is the potential to introduce "micro-prompting" technologies that can increase independence by guiding people through tasks.

Impairments with executive function may impair problem solving and make learning difficult when performing unfamiliar tasks, such as using a new washing machine. For example, a person may persevere with a strategy that does not work or be unable to keep track of the steps they have taken. Performance of familiar tasks that are habitual, such as getting dressed, can be disrupted if someone with executive difficulty fails to maintain their attention and cannot monitor their own performance. They may lose track of where they are up to in a task, and may end up repeating elements of a task or even going back to the beginning. Patient RP (Evans *et al.*, 1998), mentioned above, had difficulties of this sort in relation to bathing. She had a routine of washing her body in a particular sequence, but reported that she frequently lost track in the sequence and would keep re-starting from the beginning. This could happen many times each time she took a bath and meant that she stayed in the bath so long that it prevented her from getting to other activities on time.

Micro-prompting technologies

Micro-prompting technologies are those which guide users through a task that has several steps, or sub-tasks. For many people in many situations low-tech solutions such as simple paper-based checklists might be sufficient to support sequencing. Checklists are used as cognitive aids in many situations including medicine, aviation, and industry (Hales *et al.*, 2008) and, in everyday activities, checklists (e.g. recipes) have an important place for guiding people through tasks. The challenge for people with significant executive difficulties, however, is that it may be difficult to stay on task even with a checklist, and in this situation what is needed are intelligent systems that are able to monitor task performance and deliver appropriately timed prompts.

Two examples of intelligent micro-prompting technology, that use sensors to gather information about the environment, and respond based on this information, are GUIDE (O'Neill *et al.*, 2010) and COACH (Mihailidis *et al.*, 2008). These have been developed to aid different types of self-care.

COACH (*computer orthosis for delivering assisting activities in the home*) is a system that was initially designed to aid people with profound impairments associated with dementia to complete the task of washing hands after going to the bathroom. The system uses a sensor which detects the movement and position of the user's hands. The system then uses pattern matching and recognition algorithms to compute what steps the user is taking, and prompts them if they make any mistakes (e.g. do not use soap before drying their hands). The COACH system therefore uses technology and computing algorithms to deliver the prompts which a human caregiver would deliver if they were present. This system has been shown to be effective with several people with advanced dementia (Labelle and Mihailidis, 2006). COACH technology has been expanded to guide people through toothbrushing and is now being developed into a more interactive system to help children with autism (Boger and Mihailidis, 2011).

GUIDE is another system which attempts to help people perform self-care tasks independently. The system uses audio prompts to ask people whether or not they have performed a sub-task yet. GUIDE uses vocal feedback (yes or no answers) to decide which prompt to give next. It has been shown to improve independent prosthetic limb donning by people with vascular dementia in a within-subjects ($n = 9$) experimental design study (O'Neill *et al.*, 2010). GUIDE has also been adapted to guide people through the household and self-care tasks of the morning routine. This adaption has been shown to be useful for a person with organization difficulties following ABI – the technology improved performance on tasks such as dressing and washing in both care facility and home environments (O'Neill *et al.*, 2013).

Other innovative ideas involving guiding technology include the aQRdate system, which guides users through everyday activities using manuals on mobile phones (Gómez *et al.*, 2012). While accessing guides on a mobile phone is quite common (e.g. looking up recipes online), the innovation in this case is the use of smartphone QR (Quick Response) codes (which are matrix barcodes) that can be placed around the house in relevant locations. The user can then scan the QR code and be given a guide on how to do the household task in the vicinity of the QR code (e.g. making breakfast). This allows the prompts to be given at the right moment and in the right place. The aQRdate has been evaluated with a person with ABI and was found to reduce the amount of time they took to perform everyday tasks (Gómez *et al.*, 2012). This type of guiding system may be useful for people who find planning and organizing difficult, but it does require the user to recognize when they need to perform the household task as they have to actively scan the QR code with the smartphone.

While aQRdate uses mixed initiative planning, other devices use reactive planning to guide people to perform household tasks. Such technologies aim to sense accurately which behaviors have taken place and use this information to help people complete everyday tasks. Archipel is a system which aims to guide people through cooking tasks. Cooking tasks are particularly challenging for people with executive difficulties as they involve switching between several different tasks and keeping track of several different foods that take different times to prepare. Cooking is important for an active social life as well as being a vital household task. In Archipel sensors in the kitchen detect which items the user is interacting with. From this starting point, Archipel can learn which tasks people have particular trouble with and can determine whether somebody is having initiation, planning, attention or memory difficulties. When trialed with people with intellectual disabilities ($n = 12$), Archipel guidance was found to reduce the number of prompts the experimenters were required to give the participants during a cooking task (Bauchet *et al.*, 2009). There are other developments with tracking and sensing which could be implemented in order to predict what task the user is attempting to complete and guide them appropriately (Karg and Kirsch, 2012).

Hobbies are an important part of everyday life; however, technology has not commonly been developed to help people take up new hobbies or continue their hobbies during cognitive decline. One type of hobby for which assistive technology has been investigated is art. Hoey and colleagues describe an e-pad that guides people through computerized art-therapy tasks (Hoey *et al.*, 2010). This technology has recently been assessed with a group of older adults with mild to moderate dementia ($n = 6$). While it was found to engage users in the art task, the prompts from the device were ineffective (Leuty *et al.*, 2013).

Guiding technology is capable of helping people to do simple work-based tasks. This was demonstrated by Kirsch and colleagues when they used the COGORTH (COGnition ORTHosis) to guide somebody to perform janitorial tasks (Kirsch *et al.*, 1988). This system used a keyboard-based interaction system and gave text feedback to guide people through the task as well as visual and auditory prompts to attract attention. COGORTH was designed to be adaptable to differing levels of cognition (users could type responses to request more details, if they were able, or simply press the return key to receive the next prompt). This is important for people with executive difficulties as ability may fluctuate during the day due to fatigue, or behavioral or attentional difficulties. COGORTH was also designed to guide more than one task simultaneously, and make decisions as to which tasks should be given greater priority. These are important features for guiding people with executive difficulties in a work setting. It is rare that someone would only have to complete one task at a time during their job, and so planning and monitoring of several tasks and task switching is vital. More recently, AbleLink technology has developed PDA devices (e.g. Pocket Endeavor) which can help people with executive dysfunction to organize their day, and this may be useful in a work setting. Evidence for the efficacy of earlier forms of this technology has been gathered with people with intellectual impairment (Davies *et al.*, 2002).

Another two technologies that can help with vocational tasks have been developed by the same research team (Chang *et al.*, 2011a). Locompt uses Bluetooth to locate users and links this to a computerized guidance system. Locompt was shown to be useful at guiding two people (one with developmental difficulties and one with ABI) through a vocational food-serving task in a cafe (Chang *et al.*, 2011b). Kinept uses Kinect technology to sense people's movement and links this to a computerized guidance system. Kinept has been shown to be useful at guiding two people with task performance difficulties (one person with ABI and one person with dementia) through a pizza-making task (Chang *et al.*, 2011b). This tentative evidence shows that the prospects for using technology to help people who find it difficult to perform vocational tasks (either through executive difficulties or through other cognitive difficulties) are promising.

Smart-watches could also be a useful platform for software which could help guide people through activities in the household, help with social organization, improve uptake of hobbies and increase productivity in a working environment. Although there is no research at the moment, as this technology develops it would be interesting to see research investigating the efficacy and usability of smart-watches for guiding as well as prompting.

Barriers to technology use

Despite the research detailed above, there has been relatively little uptake of this technology among people with ABI or dementia (Evans *et al.*, 2003). Therefore, when discussing assistive technology, it is important to understand the factors which prevent and encourage people with cognitive impairment to use technology.

The factors which appear to impact on uptake of assistive technology for cognition can be split into five categories and include practical issues (e.g. cost of technology or faulty equipment), physical problems (e.g. sensory impairment which could impede technology use), cognitive impairment (e.g. the very executive functioning difficulties that technology is designed to assist may make it difficult to learn to use the technology), ethical concerns (e.g. feeling that technology is unsafe) or psychological issues (e.g. believing that using technology to compensate for abilities will prevent those abilities from naturally recovering). Each issue should be taken into account when designing technology for people with cognitive impairment.

Of these factors, cognitive impairment which is executive in nature is likely to be a particularly difficult barrier to technology uptake. A number of different executive functions are required for successful use of technology. For example, difficulties with problem solving in novel circumstances may make it challenging to use technology such as a mobile phone for the first time without a step-by-step guide. Problems with sustained attention and working memory may make it difficult to learn how to use the device. Being unable to plan in an optimal manner may mean that the device is not charged or, if it is portable, not taken when leaving the house. Impaired judgment and decision making may mean that the technology is not used at appropriate times and this may be exacerbated by poor insight into difficulties, and an associated lack of awareness of the need for, or potential value of, assistive technology. Failing to monitor navigation through the screens of a device or switch between tasks may also prevent successful use of technology. Finally, difficulties with emotional control and inhibition could lead to people becoming frustrated or angry with the device if it is challenging to master.

The potential barriers to uptake caused by executive difficulties means that it is not simply a case of "prescribing" technology for people with cognitive impairments – the nature, and severity, of the impairment must be taken into account. The idea of matching technology/user interfaces to a person's cognitive profile has rarely been touched on in the literature (for an exception, see Sutcliffe *et al.*, 2003). Furthermore, technology should be designed with the needs of the intended user group in mind. This is not only true for the function of the device (e.g. what difficulties the device is designed to help with), but also for the user interface of the device (e.g. what the device layout looks like, how the user communicates with the device, or how useful the user thinks the device will be). There are several examples in the literature of research teams developing technology by involving different user groups, for example people with dementia (Robinson *et al.*, 2009; Slegers *et al.*, 2013), people with ABI (Dawe, 2006; de Joode *et al.*, 2012), and older users (McGee-Lennon *et al.*, 2012), and this research is vital to fulfil the potential for technology to assist executive function.

Furthermore, it is very rare that someone with a degenerative disease, illness, or injury that leads to brain damage will have purely executive difficulties. Co-morbidity commonly includes poor short-term memory capacity, difficulties with attention, inability to form new memories, physical and sensory impairment, and psychological problems (e.g. lack of confidence for performing an everyday task or learning a new task may negatively impact their ability; Chan *et al.*, 2008). Technology designed to compensate for executive problems will also need to take these co-morbidities of people with executive difficulties into account.

Future innovations

Technologies which are adaptable to personal abilities, difficulties, and tastes are needed. For example, technology that has adaptable interaction modalities (e.g. via voice, touch, and so on) and multi-modal prompting (e.g. sound alerts, vibration, visual, or speech) will be useful. Wearable devices are likely to be particularly important. The arrival of Google Glass will be particularly interesting with regard to the potential for wearable, intelligent, reminding systems. Design of devices and software needs to take into account the interaction the user will have with the device, and take into account the needs of people with executive difficulties. For example, clear language, easy to follow tutorials, and functional simplicity may be desirable for people with cognitive impairments (Dawe, 2006).

It must also be recognized that some people are either unable or unwilling to interact with technology themselves (Evans *et al.*, 2003). It is still possible for technology to be of use to people in this position with the development of automated technologies that require little or no user interaction (Mihailidis *et al.*, 2011). Finally, intelligent sensing could improve the functionality of prompting or guiding devices by allowing the device to predict when and where the prompt or guide should be given. The success of such systems depends upon the number of pieces of information which sensors pick up (the more the better), the validity of the sensing (whether or not the thing being sensed actually relates to the behavior the system is making a decision on), and the accuracy of the sensing.

Conclusion

There have been numerous innovations in assistive technology over the past 20 years and, while few were specifically designed for executive dysfunction, many of them can be beneficial for people with executive functioning difficulties including lack of task initiation, difficulty switching attention, difficulty with task and social monitoring, and behavioral control and inhibition. There is a substantial evidence base for prompting technology and this functionality will become more reliable and more useful as technology improves, especially with the development of intelligent systems that are context aware. There is a small but growing literature providing evidence for the utility of guiding technologies for people who find it difficult to complete complex multi-step tasks. The advancement of intelligent sensing and decision-making algorithms will also allow guiding technologies to become more reliable and easily accessible. The design, accessibility, and availability of technology, and the extent to which it is adaptable to personal use, are important issues to be considered if the technology reported in the literature is going to be used outside of an experimental setting. Finally, clinical trials with strong methodology (including single-case experimental design studies or randomized controlled trials) are needed to move technology from clever ideas that sit on the shelves of researchers to aids that can be provided by health services.

References

Baddeley, A. D. and Wilson, B. A. (1988). Frontal Amnesia and the Dysexecutive Syndrome. *Brain and Cognition*, 7: 212–30.

Baldwin, V. N. and Powell, T. (2011). International Factors Influencing the Uptake of Memory Compensations: A Qualitative Analysis. *Neuropsychological Rehabilitation*, 21(4): 484–501.

Bauchet, J., Pigot, H., Giroux, S., Lussier-Desrochers, D., Lachapelle, Y., and Mokhtari, M. (2009). Designing Judicious Interactions for Cognitive Assistance: The Acts of Assistance Approach. In *Proceedings of the Eleventh International ACM SIGACCESS Conference on Computers and Accessibility* (pp. 11–18), Pittsburgh, PA, USA.

Boger, J. and Mihailidis, A. (2011). The Future of Intelligent Assistive Technologies for Cognition: Devices Under Development to Support Independent Living and Aging-with-Choice. *NeuroRehabilitation*, 28(3): 271–80.

Boman, I. L., Lindberg Stenvall, C., Hemmingsson, H., and Bartfai, A. (2010a). A Training Apartment with a set of Electronic Memory Aids for Patients with Cognitive Problems. *Scandinavian Journal of Occupational Therapy*, 17(2): 140–48.

Boman, I. L., Bartfai, A., Borell, L., Tham, K., and Hemmingsson, H. (2010b). Support in Everyday Activities with a Home-Based Electronic Memory Aid for Persons with Memory Impairments. *Disability and Rehabilitation: Assistive Technology*, 5(5): 339–50.

Burgess, P. W., Simons, J. S., Coates, L. M.-A., and Channon, S. (2005). The Search for Specific Planning Processes. In G. Ward and R. Morris (eds), *The Cognitive Psychology of Planning* (pp. 199–227). Hove, UK: Psychology Press.

Chan, M., Estève, D., Escriba, C., and Campo, E. (2008). A Review of Smart Homes: Present State and Future Challenges. *Computer Methods and Programs in Biomedicine*, 91(1): 55–81.

Chang, Y.-J., Chen, S.-F., and Chuang, A.-F. (2011a). A Gesture Recognition System to Transition Autonomously Through Vocational Tasks for Individuals with Cognitive Impairments. *Research in Developmental Disabilities*, 32(6): 2064–68.

Chang, Y.-J., Wang, T.-Y., and Chen, Y.-R. (2011b). A Location-Based Prompting System to Transition Autonomously Through Vocational Tasks for Individuals with Cognitive Impairments. *Research in Developmental Disabilities*, 32(6): 2669–73.

Chu, Y., Chol Song, Y., Levinson, R., and Kautz, H. (2012). Interactive Activity Recognition and Prompting to Assist People with Cognitive Disabilities. *Journal of Ambient Intelligence and Smart Environments*, 4(5): 443–59.

Davies, D. K., Stock, S. E., and Wehmeyer, M. L. (2002). Enhancing Independent Time-Management Skills of Individuals with Mental Retardation using a Palmtop Personal Computer. *Mental Retardation*, 40(5): 358–65.

Dawe, M. (2006). Desperately Seeking Simplicity: How Young Adults with Cognitive Disabilities and Their Families Adopt Assistive Technologies. In *CHI 2006 Proceedings* (pp. 1143–52), Montreal, Canada.

De Joode, E., Van Heugten, C., Verhey, F., and Van Boxtel, M. (2010). Efficacy and Usability of Assistive Technology for Patients with Cognitive Deficits: A Systematic Review. *Clinical Rehabilitation*, 24(8): 701–14.

De Joode, E., Proot, I., Slegers, K., Van Heugten, C., Verhey, F., and Van Boxtel, M. (2012). The use of Standard Calendar Software by Individuals with Acquired Brain Injury and Cognitive Complaints: A Mixed Methods Study. *Disability and Rehabilitation. Assistive Technology*, 7(5): 389–98.

De Joode, E., Van Heugten, C. M., Verhey, F. R. J., and Van Boxtel, M. P. J. (2013). Effectiveness of an Electronic Cognitive Aid in Patients with Acquired Brain Injury: A Multicentre Randomised Parallel-Group Study. *Neuropsychological Rehabilitation*, 23(1): 133–56.

Delis, D. C., Kaplan, E., and Kramer, J. H. (2001). *Delis-Kaplan Executive Function System (D-KEFS)*. Antonio, TX: Psychological Corporation.

Dowds, M. M., Lee, P. H., Sheer, J. B., O'Neil-Pirozzi, T. M., Xenopoulos-Oddsson, A., Goldstein, R., and Glenn, M. B. (2011). Electronic Reminding Technology Following Traumatic Brain Injury: Effects on Timely Task Completion. *The Journal of Head Trauma Rehabilitation*, 26(5): 339–47.

Emslie, H., Wilson, B. A., Quirk, K., Evans, J. J., and Watson, P. (2007). Using a Paging System in the Rehabilitation of Encephalitic Patients. *Neuropsychological Rehabilitation*, 17(4–5): 567–81.

Evans, J. J., Emslie, H., and Wilson, B. A. (1998). External Cueing Systems in the Rehabilitation of Executive Impairments of Action. *Journal of the International Neuropsychological Society*, 4(04): 399–408.

Evans, J. J., Wilson, B. A., Needham, P., and Brentnall, S. (2003). Who Makes Good Use of Memory Aids? Results of a Survey of People with Acquired Brain Injury. *Journal of the International Neuropsychological Society*, 9(6): 925–35.

Fish, J., Evans, J. J., Nimmo, M., Martin, E., Kersel, D., Bateman, A., and Manly, T. (2007). Rehabilitation of Executive Dysfunction Following Brain Injury: "Content-Free"

Cueing Improves Everyday Prospective Memory Performance. *Neuropsychologia*, 45(6): 1318–30.

Fish, J., Manly, T., Emslie, H., Evans, J. J., and Wilson, B. A. (2008). Compensatory Strategies for Acquired Disorders of Memory and Planning: Differential Effects of a Paging System for Patients with Brain Injury of Traumatic Versus Cerebrovascular Aetiology. *Journal of Neurology, Neurosurgery and Psychiatry*, 79(8): 930–35.

Gillespie, A., Best, C., and O'Neill, B. (2012). Cognitive Function and Assistive Technology for Cognition: A Systematic Review. *Journal of the International Neuropsychological Society*, 18(01): 1–19.

Gómez, J., Montoro, G., Haya, P. A., Alamán, X., Alves, S., and Martínez, M. (2012). Adaptive Manuals as Assistive Technology to Support and Train People with Acquired Brain Injury in their Daily Life Activities. *Personal and Ubiquitous Computing*, 17(6): 1117–26.

Hales, B., Terblanche, M., Fowler, R., and Sibbald, W. (2008). Development of Medical Checklists for Improved Quality of Patient Care. *International Journal for Quality in Health Care: Journal of the International Society for Quality in Health Care/ISQua*, 20(1): 22–30.

Hayes, T. L., Cobbinah, K., Dishongh, T., Kaye, J. A., Kimel, J., Labhard, M., and Vurgun, S. (2009). A Study of Medication-Taking and Unobtrusive, Intelligent Reminding. *Telemedicine Journal and e-Health: The Official Journal of the American Telemedicine Association*, 15(8): 770–76.

Hoey, J., Zutis, K., Leuty, V., and Mihailidis, A. (2010). A Tool to Promote Prolonged Engagement in Art Therapy: Design and Development from Arts Therapist Requirements. In *Proceedings of the 12th International ACM SIGACCESS Conference on Computers and Accessibility*, October (pp. 211–18).

Jamieson, M., Cullen, B., McGee-Lennon, M., Brewster, S., and Evans, J. J. (2014). The Efficacy of Cognitive Prosthetic Technology for People with Memory Impairments: A Systematic Review And Meta-Analysis. *Neuropsychological Rehabilitation*, 24(3–4): 419–44.

Karg, M. and Kirsch, A. (2012). Acquisition and Use of Transferable, Spatio-Temporal Plan Representations for Human–Robot Interaction. In *Intelligent Robots and Systems (IROS), IEEE/RSJ International Conference*, October (pp. 5220–26).

Kirsch, N., Levine, S., Lajiness, R., Mossaro, M., Schneider, M., and Donders, J. (1988). Improving Functional Performance with Computerized Task Guidance Systems. In *ICAART 88* (pp. 564–66), Montreal, Canada.

Labelle, K.-L. and Mihailidis, A. (2006). The Use of Automated Prompting to Facilitate Handwashing in Persons with Dementia. *The American Journal of Occupational Therapy: Official Publication of the American Occupational Therapy Association*, 60(4): 442–50.

Lemoncello, R., Sohlberg, M. M., Fickas, S., and Prideaux, J. (2011a). A Randomised Controlled Crossover Trial Evaluating Television Assisted Prompting (TAP) for Adults with Acquired Brain Injury. *Neuropsychological Rehabilitation*, 21(6): 825–46.

Lemoncello, R., Sohlberg, M. M., Fickas, S., Albin, R., and Harn, B. E. (2011b). Phase I Evaluation of the Television Assisted Prompting System to increase Completion of Home Exercises Among Stroke Survivors. *Disability and Rehabilitation. Assistive Technology*, 6(5): 440–52.

Leuty, V., Boger, J., Young, L., Hoey, J., and Mihailidis, A. (2013). Engaging Older Adults with Dementia in Creative Occupations using Artificially Intelligent Assistive Technology. *Assistive Technology*, 25(2): 72–9.

Levinson, R. (1997). The Planning and Execution Assistant and Trainer (PEAT). *The Journal of Head Trauma Rehabilitation*, 12(2): 85–91.

McDonald, A., Haslam, C., Yates, P., Gurr, B., Leeder, G., and Sayers, A. (2011). Google Calendar: A New Memory Aid to Compensate for Prospective Memory Deficits Following Acquired Brain Injury. *Neuropsychological Rehabilitation*, 21(6): 784–807.

McGee-Lennon, M., Smeaton, A., and Brewster, S. (2012). Designing Home Care Reminder Systems: Lessons Learned Through Co-Design with Older Users. In *6th International Conference on Pervasive Computing Technologies for Healthcare (PervasiveHealth)*, *2012*, May (pp. 49–56). Los Alamitos, CA: IEEE.

Mihailidis, A., Boger, J. N., Craig, T., and Hoey, J. (2008). The COACH Prompting System to Assist Older Adults with Dementia Through Handwashing: An Efficacy Study. *BMC Geriatrics*, 8(1): 28.

Mihailidis, A., Boger, J., Hoey, J., and Jiancaro, T. (2011). Zero Effort Technologies: Considerations, Challenges and Use in Health, Wellness and Rehabilitation. *Synthesis Lectures on Assistive, Rehabilitative and Health-Preserving Technologies*, 1(2): 1–94.

Miyake, A. and Shah, P. (eds) (1999). *Models of Working Memory: Mechanisms of Active Maintenance and Executive Control*. Cambridge, UK: Cambridge University Press.

Miyake, A., Friedman, N. P., Emerson, M. J., Witzki, A. H., Howerter, A., and Wager, T. D. (2000). The Unity and Diversity of Executive Functions and their Contributions to Complex "Frontal Lobe" Tasks: A Latent Variable Analysis. *Cognitive Psychology*, 41(1): 49–100.

Norman, D. A. and Shallice, T. (1986). *Attention to Action* (pp. 1–18). New York, NY: Springer.

O'Neill, B., Moran, K., and Gillespie, A. (2010). Scaffolding Rehabilitation Behaviour using a Voice-Mediated Assistive Technology for Cognition. *Neuropsychological Rehabilitation*, 20(4): 509–27.

O'Neill, B., Best, C., Gillespie, A., and O'Neill, L. (2013). Automated Prompting Technologies in Rehabilitation and at Home. *Social Care and Neurodisability*, 4(1): 17–28.

Pollack, M. E., Brown, L., Colbry, D., McCarthy, C. E., Orosz, C., Peintner, B., and Tsamardinos, I. (2003). Autominder: An Intelligent Cognitive Orthotic System for People with Memory Impairment. *Robotics and Autonomous Systems*, 44(3–4): 273–82.

Rashidi, P. and Mihailidis, A. (2013) A Survey on Ambient-Assisted Living Tools for Older Adults. IEEE *Journal of Biomedical Health Information*, 17: 579–90.

Robinson, L., Brittain, K., Lindsay, S., Jackson, D., and Olivier, P. (2009). Keeping In Touch Everyday (KITE) Project: Developing Assistive Technologies with People with Dementia and their Carers to Promote Independence. *International Psychogeriatrics/IPA*, 21(3): 494–502.

Roth, R. M., Isquith, P. K., and Gioia, G. A. (2014). Assessment of Executive Functioning Using the Behavior Rating Inventory of Executive Function (BRIEF). In S. Goldstein and J. A. Naglieri (eds), *Handbook of Executive Functioning*. New York, NY: Springer.

Shallice, T. and Burgess, P. (1991). Higher-Order Cognitive Impairments and Frontal Lobe Lesions in Man. In H. S. Levin, H. M. Eisenberg, and A. L. Benton (eds), *Frontal Lobe Function and Dysfunction* (pp. 125–38). New York: Oxford University Press.

Simpson, R., Schreckenghost, D., LoPresti, E. F., and Kirsch, N. (2006). Plans and Planning in Smart Homes. In *Designing Smart Homes* (pp. 71–84). Berlin, Heidelberg: Springer.

Slegers, K., Wilkinson, A., and Hendriks, N. (2013). Active Collaboration in Healthcare Design: Participatory Design to Develop a Dementia Care App. In *CHI '13 Extended Abstracts on Human Factors in Computing Systems*, April (pp. 475–80). New York, NY: ACM.

Snoek, J., Hoey, J., Stewart, L., Zemel, R. S., and Mihailidis, A. (2009). Automated Detection of Unusual Events on Stairs. *Image and Vision Computing*, 27(1–2): 153–66.

Stapleton, S., Adams, M., and Atterton, L. (2007). A Mobile Phone as a Memory Aid for Individuals with Traumatic Brain Injury: A Preliminary Investigation. *Brain Injury*, 21(4): 401–11.

Stuss, D. T. and Knight, R. T. (eds) (2013). *Principles of Frontal Lobe Function*. Oxford, UK: Oxford University Press.

Sutcliffe, A., Fickas, S., Ehlhardt, L. A., and Sohlberg, M. M. (2003). Investigating the Usability of Assistive User Interfaces. *Interacting with Computers*, 15(4): 577–602.

Van Den Broek, M. D., Downes, J., Johnson, Z., Dayus, B., and Hilton, N. (2000). Evaluation of an Electronic Memory Aid in the Neuropsychological Rehabilitation of Prospective Memory Deficits. *Brain Injury*, 14(5): 455–62.

Van Hulle, A. and Hux, K. (2006). Improvement Patterns Among Survivors of Brain Injury: Three Case Examples Documenting the Effectiveness of Memory Compensation Strategies. *Brain Injury*, 20(1): 101–09.

Wilson, B. A., Evans, J. J., Alderman, N., Burgess, P. W., and Emslie, H. (1997). Behavioural Assessment of the Dysexecutive Syndrome. In P. Rabbitt (ed.), *Methodology of Frontal and Executive Function* (pp. 239–50). Hove, UK: Psychology Press Ltd.

Wilson, B. A., Emslie, H. C., Quirk, K., and Evans, J. J. (2001). Reducing Everyday Memory and Planning Problems by Means of a Paging System: A Randomised Control Crossover Study. *Journal of Neurology, Neurosurgery and Psychiatry*, 70(4): 477–82.

7

COGNITIVE SUPPORT FOR LANGUAGE AND SOCIAL INTERACTION

Norman Alm

A number of technological supports have been developed for people whose physical impairments make it impossible for them to speak. These physical impairments still severely impede the rate at which the person can communicate, even with technical help. Research efforts are ongoing to find ways in which the conversational momentum can be improved given such a low input rate. A number of prototypes have been developed and evaluated that involve pre-storing conversational material in various structures. To the extent that these structures are derived from our understanding of the cognitive underpinnings of communicative acts, they can be seen as rudimentary cognitive prostheses. In order to be of assistance to people whose communication difficulties are cognitive ones, such systems will need to act as active prompts as well as passive storage containers for language units.

The importance of conversational interaction

Being able to communicate is the essence of being human. Our ability to use language is a primary skill employed in social interaction, and we are a social species. Mothers begin conversing with babies from birth with a form of language that familiarizes them with the rhythms of spoken interchange (Shore, 1997). As growing children we constantly learn about the world, both physical and social, through conversation. We are socialized through talk, and continue to make our way in the world largely through interpersonal communication (Beattie, 1983: 2).

Being non-speaking, while cognitively still intact, can result from brain damage at birth (cerebral palsy), or progressive conditions such as motor neurone disease. The impact this has on the person has been described eloquently by one author who was non-speaking through cerebral palsy: "If I were granted one wish and one wish only, I would not hesitate for an instant to request that I be able to talk, if only for one day, or even one hour" (Sienkiewicz-Mercer and Kaplan, 1989).

Communication tools for non-speaking people

Technology has been developed to assist those with physical impairments to communicate. People with a congenital or acquired inability to control the organs of speech, but who are otherwise cognitively unimpaired, are able to make use of computer-produced speech controlled by specially designed interfaces. Such systems are a form of what is termed Augmentative and Alternative Communication (AAC).

A problem that all these systems share is the slow output of speech that it is possible to produce. If an able-bodied professional typist were to provide input for an AAC system, they would manage about 50–80 words per minute. Even this is slow compared to speech, which averages about 150–180 words per minute. A typical AAC user, however, has a lack of fine physical control, which is why they cannot control the organs of speech. This slows their communication rate down to about 2–15 words per minute (Beukelman and Mirenda, 2005).

Utterance-based systems

Attempts have been made to speed up speech output in such systems by developing prototypes whose unit of expression is not a letter or a word, but an entire utterance. The goal has been to try to duplicate the speed and effectiveness of unimpaired communication by outputting more words per activation (Todman et al., 2008; Arnott and Alm, 2013). Utterance-based communication support systems have been experimented with, usually involving pre-stored text, with utterances organized in a variety of ways. The hope has been that ways could be found to supply appropriate utterances easily, and to some extent be able to predict likely next utterances. Organizing approaches that have been examined include sets of phatic expressions, feedback remarks, hypertext, frames, scripts, and narratives.

Phatic interaction

Phatic interaction is interaction whose purpose is not the conveying of external information, but tasks that relate to the interaction itself, such as ritualized greeting and farewell routines (Laver, 1981). The opening and closing stages of conversations are particularly formulaic and relatively predictable parts of an interaction (Krivonos and Knapp, 1975; Laver, 1981; Schegloff and Sacks, 1973). A prototype called CHAT (Conversation Helped by Automatic Talk) was designed to contain recognizable and formulaic stages of conversation such as greetings, responses to greetings, small talk, wrap-up remarks, and farewells, hence accommodating the opening and closing phases of conversation (Alm et al., 1987; Alm et al., 1992). Utterances were stored in the system to fulfill these conversational stages in sufficient numbers to allow the system to randomize its selection of appropriate utterances within individual stages, in order to avoid frequent repetition.

Backchannels (feedback remarks)

Backchannel (feedback) communication is important in maintaining and controlling the flow of conversation, and in giving the speaker an indication of how the listener is feeling about the conversation (Yngve, 1970). Backchannels are short feedback words, phrases, or sounds. They are normally delivered overlapping the utterances of the other speaker and, far from creating an interruption, they actually assist the other speaker to carry on by conveying reactions to what they are saying.

The CHAT prototype also contained a set of general purpose backchannel remarks (e.g. "Uh-huh," "Okay," "Great!" and "That's too bad") which could be output quickly. Timely production of this sort of communication is essential for it to be effective. Generic utterances (Ball *et al.*, 1999) and formulaic utterances (Wray, 2001) such as these gave the system a certain degree of flexibility and variability for use in conversation. The prototype thus allowed the user to open a conversation, to give feedback to remarks from the other speaker, and to close the conversation, all with the phrases produced rapidly, even with a motor impairment. Trials of CHAT showed average speaking rates of 54 words per minute (Alm *et al.*, 1992). Conversation was restricted to greeting, responding, giving feedback, and parting, of course, which only covers a part of conversation. However, participants judged the experience as more pleasant, natural, and easy than attempting the same communication using their standard AAC system.

Hypertext

Having established that pre-stored text had a role to play in the more formulaic aspects of conversation, the next step in the research was to explore methods for storing and retrieving larger amounts of conversational material. A priority here was to retain an easy-to-use user interface that did not require a large effort from the user in order to produce appropriate texts. An ideal system would produce a form of conversational prediction that would be able to produce automatically appropriate choices for the next thing to say.

Hypertext was proposed by one research group as a structure that could facilitate this type of predictive system, since hypertext is a method for storing and navigating through information using highly flexible associative links (Alm *et al.*, 1990). Any cross-referencing in documents can be considered as a simple form of hypertext, but the provision of a rich network of such associations on a computer with interactive capabilities gives hypertext its real character. Hypertext thus might be able to model the flexible way in which the mind stores and recalls conversation items, and the way in which conversational items are introduced into a dialogue in such a way that maintains the coherence of the conversation.

The problem of getting lost in a hypertext structure suggests that it might be a more suitable environment for browsing than for directed information finding. There is an interesting parallel here with the way informal conversation wanders through a number of topics, much as a user might browse through a richly connected information system. There may be a trade-off between effectiveness and ease of use where hypertext is being used to convey information. Where hypertext is being used as a store for conversational material through which a user is allowed, and in fact, encouraged, to "wander," this would not be as much of a problem.

The difficulty with actually producing a hypertext-based communication system was that the links between stored text segments would need to be coded individually. The enormous overhead this would involve for a system which included a large number of texts initially seemed to rule out a practical application of this idea. More recently, a simplified hypermedia system based on a touchscreen was developed to assist people with dementia to communicate. By reducing the number of links per screen, but retaining a degree of richness in the material presented, a workable system was created. The idea was to have a simple interface that gave access to a set of items that were picked at random from a very large store (Alm *et al.*, 2007). The system is described later in this chapter.

Frames

Data structures that can be used to represent stereotypical situations have also been used for pre-stored candidate utterances. When one encounters a new situation one can be seen as selecting from memory a re-usable framework which can be adapted to fit the current situation by changing details as necessary. A frame is a data-structure for representing a stereotypical situation, such as being in a certain kind of shop, or going to a dance. A frame can have variables, called slots, which then can account for a variety of individual circumstances. (Minsky, 1975).

A prototype AAC system, Frametalker, has been constructed using the frame concept. This work was based on the view that talk is a type of action, and action can be represented, and interpreted, in a holistic fashion with respect to the context in which it is used (Higginbotham *et al.*, 2000). Utterance templates were devised, which were stored in frames with slots being used for the insertion of different items from a database, thus giving a flexible tool for the generation of individual utterances for use in context during conversation. Word rates of more than 40 words per minute were achieved by participants during trials with Frametalker (Higginbotham *et al.*, 2002).

Scripts

Transactional interactions, which are interactions aimed at achieving particular tasks, such as placing an order for a meal in a restaurant or consulting a physician, can be seen as relatively formulaic and therefore somewhat predictable. As with previous examples, formulaic or predictable features in communication can be advantageous to a communications system user. Script, or schema, approaches have been investigated as a way of applying anticipated sequences and structures to trans-actional interactions such that the system would retrieve and make available appro-priate and relevant utterances for each stage of a particular interaction (Alm *et al.*, 1995; Vanderheyden, 1995; Carpenter *et al.*, 1997; Harper *et al.*, 1998).

Scripts have also been used by people without disabilities in situations where there is not enough time to stop and consider a change of plan, such as when piloting a high-performance combat aircraft. In this case, a plan is devised before the flight for the pilot to follow. If the pilot encounters a situation completely different from what was expected, instead of working out a way of departing from the script they may just have to return to base and devise a new script (Amalberti and Valot, 1993). This is an interesting example of what Newell has described as the ordinary/extraordinary concept: the same technology that helps ordinary people to perform extraordinary tasks (high workload, environmentally unfriendly) may be used by extraordinary peo-ple who need the technology to accomplish ordinary tasks (Newell, 1995).

As with frames, scripts were originally proposed as a way to give "intelligence" to an artificial system, such as a question answering program, or a robot (Schank and Abelson, 1977). Both frames and scripts came up against the problem of the rich-ness and variety of real life, which required an unsatisfactory series of add-ons and adjustments that relegated these ideas to seemingly valid but over-ambitious approaches. The situation with AAC was quite different from trying to build an autonomous robot or interviewing system. With AAC, there is a person in charge of the technology, who can steer it. What is needed is not a fully autonomous sys-tem, but a tool that can add momentum to the slow and limited input controls possible for a user with physical impairments (Alm *et al.*, 1992).

Applying this idea to AAC, scripts might be created for the person to use to achieve particular tasks, such as shopping, visiting a doctor, or ordering food. A prototype AAC script system with six scripts was developed in one research project. The scripts were: in the restaurant, shopping, at the doctor, around home, on the phone, and chatting. These scripts were derived from the suggestions of a focus group of AAC users who provided input for the research project. They were situations in which they would like to able to negotiate without the help of another person, which currently was not possible. The prototype was shown to be effective in a limited number of trials; however, it became clear that a larger repertoire of scripts was required for more general application of the concept. An authoring system was then devised, which allowed the person, with the aid of caregivers, to craft their own scripts. The amount of time and effort involved in this, and the knowledge of conversational patterns needed, meant that the system was in fact not popular (Dye *et al.*, 1998).

Narrative

An important part of social interaction is telling stories to each other. These may be long narratives, but commonly are short descriptions of something that has happened that we want to share. Relating your past experiences provides a way of sharing these with others and also portraying the sort of person you are (Quasthoff and Nikolaus, 1982). Building up a personal story-base plays an important part in an individual's social and educational development. Telling and retelling, framing and reframing personal stories helps us to reflect on our life and share our reflections with others. Stories provide one person's views on the meaning of their experiences, and actually help to form the person's sense of self (Polkinghorne, 1995).

Methods have been developed to provide AAC users with better access to narrative conversation. Research projects have used technology to support interactional story-telling. Story-telling tools, including ways to introduce a story, tell it at an appropriate pace, and respond with feedback to listeners' comments, have been developed (Waller, 2006).

Different types of narrative have been explored, including joke telling. The STANDUP system used artificial intelligence techniques to generate completely novel puns for non-speaking children to enjoy using. Evaluation of the system with children with cerebral palsy showed that participants were able to use it successfully to generate novel puns (O'Mara and Waller, 2003; Waller et al., 2009).

The use of multimedia broadens the scope for narrative and floor-holding available to the non-speaking person, helping them to engage a conversation partner in attending to audio-visual material as part of a conversation. Photographs can be used in story-telling (Balabanović et al., 2000) and video recordings can provide a means for illustrating personal histories and narratives (Hine and Arnott, 2002; Hine et al., 2003).

The emerging technologies of "smart environments" and natural language generation have been used in a narrative generation system to allow non-speaking school children to tell their parents what happened at school that day. Sensors provided information about the child's movements through the school and their encounters with staff. This data was fed into a natural language generation algorithm that created conversation utterances about what had happened that the child could then output from their speech synthesizer to share the news of their day with family when they got home (Black et al., 2010).

Modeling conversational structure

The aim of all the utterance-based supported communication, as described above, is to try to enable a person who uses AAC to produce appropriate utterances at the right time for use in conversation. For this, a model of the conversation can provide "scaffolding," by means of which the AAC system can make a best attempt to provide appropriate conversational utterances for the non-speaking person to use during live conversation. It is necessary for this to be achieved in real-time as far as possible, without significant delays.

In addition to the partial models of conversation described above (phatics and feedback remarks, hypertext, frames, scripts, and narratives), a number of attempts have been made to create an overall model of conversation that would be helpful in designing AAC systems. One existing attempt at a comprehensive model of unimpaired conversation was examined as a possible source of a model for AAC conversations, but was found to be more suggestive than exhaustive in the categories it proposed, and to have a number of gaps (Wang, 2005).

Another line of research similarly took as a starting point the work of the conversation analysts (e.g. Garfinkel, 1967; Sacks *et al.*, 1974; Levinson, 1983), the systemic functional linguists (Halliday, 1985), and the synthesizing of much of this work by Clark (Clark, 1996).

The first attempt at an overall conversational model for an AAC system noted that most conversations proceeded in these stages: greetings, response to greeting, small talk, main section of conversation, wrap-ups, farewells (Alm *et al.*, 1987, 1992). Another proposed model foregrounded the pragmatics of conversation; that is, the personal and interactional goals which the participants want to achieve. For instance, achieving the goal of creating a good impression of yourself will be aided by maintaining a good conversational flow, which can be assisted by the use of pre-stored phrases as opposed to creating phrases from words or letters (Todman and Alm, 2003). More recently, a model has been proposed which tries to account both for speakers and also their physical and social environment. This is a highly ambitious proposal, and the model so far is at a high level of abstraction. It will be a further task to fill in the lower level details (Hedvall and Rydeman, 2010, 2011). A useful summary of the work thus far in overall conversational modeling for AAC can be found in (Arnott and Alm, 2013).

From supporting conversation to prompting it

The systems described so far were developed originally for people who face physical impairments that do not allow them to speak, but who are cognitively intact. The challenge has been to devise systems which are easily used, but which convey what the user wants to say quickly, ideally approaching the speed of unimpeded speech. The aim is to increase the momentum of conversation by providing more output for minimal input (Alm *et al.*, 1992). As part of this effort, structures for storing and retrieving large amounts of conversational material were developed. One criticism made of this approach at the time was that having such material available would tend to prompt the user to employ what was easily in front of them rather than say precisely but laboriously what they wanted to, crafting an utterance from scratch. The pre-stored text systems might prompt the user in ways that pre-empted their control over the conversational direction.

This is a valid concern, but raising it interestingly suggested a new direction such systems might take. Since these conversational tools and models, as well as being passive structures to hold material for the user, could also be used as a source of prompts for what the user might like to say next, a new application that suggested itself was assisting people whose communication block was not physical, but cognitive.

Aphasia

Aphasia is impaired comprehension or production of language, most commonly caused by a stroke which affects an area of brain involved in these activities. A communication support system for people with aphasia, called Lingraphica, has been developed based on accessing language through pictures, icons, and scenes depicting everyday objects and activities (Steele *et al.*, 1989; Steele, 2004). Here, the person's inability to produce an utterance is circumvented by giving them access to a visual representation of words and phrases. This can act as a substitute for speech, or as a helpful prompt.

Following on from some of the work on structured storage of conversational material described in the previous sections, a prototype, called TalksBack, was developed to be of help for people with aphasia, by using a structure to actively prompt the user as to what they might like to say next. The structure was based on information about the user and the person they were speaking with, their relationship, the topic being discussed, and the user's intention; that is, the speech act they wished to employ. The set of possible topics was modeled using a semantic network, so that the system "knew" that if the conversation was about pets, a suitable next topic might be something else about the family and not, say, a political point. The idea of modeling the user and communication partners was to help guide the topic selection. Having the user's relationship with the other person was useful so that, for instance, if the user was talking with a friend and wished to tell a joke, the system would search for a pre-stored joke that would be appropriate to tell (if the user were speaking with their mother, a different joke might be chosen!). In small-scale trials, the system was found to give the person with aphasia more control of the conversation, and increased the length of their utterances (Broumley, 1994; Waller *et al.*, 1998).

Dementia

Dementia is the term used for a serious loss of key cognitive abilities. In older people, the primary cause of dementia is Alzheimer's Disease, and the second most common cause is a stroke or multiple strokes. Affected cognitive functions include memory – particularly working (short-term) memory, attention, language, and problem-solving ability.

One of the most distressing aspects of dementia is the inability to carry out even the simplest conversation with a relative or caregiver. Without short-term memory, people with dementia tend to repeat themselves endlessly and are unable to participate in a conversation. However, even in severely affected people, their long-term memories can be relatively well preserved. If the person can be prompted about these memories, they are able to enjoy relating events from their past. Although it is possible for someone who is well-acquainted with the person's past to guide them towards their long-term memories and support them in telling their stories, it is hard work. It is very difficult for a relative or caregiver to have a relaxed and mutually enjoyable conversation with the person who has dementia.

A multidisciplinary team of psychologists, designers, and software engineers have developed a system called CIRCA, which supports communication in dementia. CIRCA is touchscreen-based and takes over from the caregiver the job of prompting and supporting the communication of a person with dementia. Its aim was to restore the ability of the person with dementia to have satisfying interactions with relatives, friends, and caregivers (Alm *et al.*, 2004).

CIRCA consists of a large collection of generic reminiscence material, drawn from a number of media archives. The content consists of photographs, film clips, and music. The material is arranged in a hypermedia format, so it can be navigated flexibly, following and prompting a natural conversational flow. As suggested in the section on hypertext above, this structure can allow for a natural conversational progression, with the participants able to output one utterance and then move to one of a range of suitable next utterances.

CIRCA was shown in evaluations to be superior to traditional reminiscence sessions with scrapbooks and other memorabilia, which are time-consuming to assemble and a chore to deliver. The system has also been shown to restore a degree of conversational control to the person with dementia, which is an effect not seen with traditional methods. One surprising finding was that generic reminiscence material from public archives was better at eliciting a wide range of personal reminiscences than personal material. This is because the personal material tended to prompt exactly the same story each time. With a very large collection of generic material, the chances of prompting a wide range of stories was increased. In fact, it was commonly observed that stories were unearthed that the family had not heard before (Alm *et al.*, 2007; Astell *et al.*, 2010a; Astell *et al.*, 2010b).

Distributed cognition

A new challenge for developing communication support systems that model cognitive processes will be to acknowledge the finding that it is helpful to view cognition as distributed and not as simply located within the mind of an individual. Distributed cognition as an approach posits that knowledge lies not only within the individual but also resides in their social and external environment. The field had its start from the influential work of Hutchins, who argued that "cognition is a fundamentally cultural process" (Hutchins, 1995: 374). When a group is performing a task, different cognitive aspects of the event may be performed by different group members. The external environment can also play a part in a cognitive process. For instance, the placement of objects in an office can act as a memory prompt for the occupant.

Related to this chapter, but also to the whole message of this book, is the fact that the proliferation of electronic and computer-based aids to computation, information providing, and communication have to some degree expanded the definition of cognitive activities to include these artifacts (see O'Neill and Gillespie, Chapter 1, this volume). For communication support systems, this suggests a number of new directions.

For cognition distributed across members of a group, it might be possible to develop ways in which both (or all) participants in an encounter could equally make use of the technology, so that the conversation is, as happens with unimpaired communication, "co-constructed." As Clark puts it: "Contributing to a discourse [...] appears to require more than just uttering the right words at the right time. It seems to consist of collective acts performed by the participants working together" (Clark and Schaefer, 1989: 259).

Work has been done on including the communication partner in constructing the augmented communicator's output (Higginbotham *et al.*, 2007). Using speech recognition has also been explored as a way of automatically capturing the contribution of a naturally speaking partner so that the information can be used by the communications system in selecting candidate utterances for the non-speaking participant (Wisenburn and Higginbotham, 2008, 2009).

In an interesting application of AAC principles outside of AAC, a prototype system was developed for cross-language communication that was inspired by AAC systems. This prototype took the unusual approach of having both users equally accessing a large store of utterances organized into openers and closers, scripts, tables, and feedback remarks. The idea was that both participants were in fact "speech impaired" in that they could not speak or understand the other person's language. The interface was designed for a touchscreen, and presented the material to each user in their own language, switching back and forth as each person took their turn (Iwabuchi *et al.*, 2001). It may be possible to take this idea further, with the starting point being that interacting with language may be seen as a type of game (Wittgenstein, 1953). One research direction would be to examine to what extent a third element to the communication, which could have some of the characteristics of a game, and which was designed to be controlled equally efficiently by the non-speaking person and the communication partner, would be acceptable and capable of creating a satisfying interaction.

It would be useful to devise ways that a communication support system could include awareness of the social context of the encounter to produce appropriate candidate utterances for the user (Hedvall and Rydeman, 2010, 2011). This was tried out with the TalksBack prototype, but involved a helper entering all the required information beforehand, in consultation with the user.

For cognition that includes our external environment, we could devise ways that a communication support system could include awareness of the external context of the encounter to produce appropriate candidate utterances for the user. One researcher has proposed that an AAC user would find it very useful, if, on approaching a supermarket, the supermarket would make available a set of vocabulary and phrases useful for shopping there, which the AAC user could download as they entered (K. Nakamura, personal communication, 2007).

Some work has suggested using the Internet as a source of conversational material for use in an AAC system (Ashraf and Ricketts, 2003; Reiter *et al.*, 2009; Luo *et al.*, 2007). The idea is that the person using AAC would be able to say something like, "What did you think of the game last night?", where the phrase "What did you think of" would be a template and the phrase "the game last night" plus accompanying material would be produced from information accessed on the Internet and then analyzed for use. The subsequent conversation would proceed with the AAC user making use of a series of such templates with slots and newly created fillers for the slots derived from Internet news sites and similar sources. The challenges will lie in how to harvest such material effectively and efficiently, how to process it, and how to present it to the person using AAC for easy inclusion in their conversation.

Physical context awareness is also technically feasible. Tiny low-cost sensors can create an environment that is continuously monitoring itself. RFID (radio frequency identification) tags are small devices that can be attached to objects and which allow the object to broadcast information about itself to anyone nearby. Sensor networks and pervasive technology can be used to detect a person's presence and movement in spaces (Gil *et al.*, 2007) and their interactions with objects. Such technology is moving us towards what has been called "the internet of things," potentially a global network of physical objects as pervasive and as ubiquitous as the worldwide web itself. As described above, a system has been developed using a "smart environment" to feed in information about a disabled school pupil's movements through the school to enable them to tell the story of their day when they get home (Black *et al.*, 2010).

Even from these initial speculative studies, it seems that applying the concept of distributed cognition to the problem of augmented communication has the capacity to improve its effectiveness and impact. Bringing to bear information from the environment and from other participants in the interaction has the potential not only to provide much needed assistance for the hard-pressed non-speaking person, but to more accurately reflect the nature of conversational communication "in the wild."

Conclusion

We have seen that a number of inventive approaches have been taken to providing better communicational support for severely physically impaired non-speaking people. By viewing such prototypes as sources of prompts as well as just being structures for storing communicational content, we might have a starting point for developing cognitive supports for communication. Promising results have been reported for such systems supporting communication for people with aphasia and dementia. The concept of distributed cognition may provide new insights and approaches to proving this much needed support for a wide variety of people whose communicative problems are cognitive in origin.

References

Alm, N., Newell, A. F., and Arnott, J. L. (1987). A Communication Aid which Models Conversational Patterns. *Proceedings of the 10th Annual Conference on Rehabilitation Technology*, June 19–23 (pp. 127–29), San Jose, CA.

Alm, N., Arnott, J. L., and Newell, A. F. (1990). Hypertext as a Host for an Augmentative Communication System. *Proceedings of the European Conference on the Advancement of Rehabilitation Technology. ECART* (pp. 14.4a–14.4b). Maastricht, the Netherlands: Institute for Rehabilitation Research.

Alm, N., Arnott, J. L., and Newell A. F. (1992). Prediction and Conversational Momentum in an Augmentative Communication System. *Communications of the ACM*, 35(5): 46–57.

Alm, N., Morrison, A., and Arnott, J. L. (1995). A Communication System based on Scripts, Plans and Goals for Enabling Non-speaking People to Conduct Telephone Conversations. *Proceedings of the IEEE Conference on Systems, Man and Cybernetics*, October 22–25 (Vol. 3, pp. 2408–12), Vancouver, BC, Canada.

Alm, N., Ellis, M., Astell, A., Dye, R., Gowans, G., and Campbell, J. (2004). A Cognitive Prosthesis and Communication Support for People with Dementia. *Neuropsychological Rehabilitation*, 14(1/2): 117–34.

Alm, N., Dye, R., Gowans, G., Campbell, J., Astell, A., and Ellis, M. (2007). A Communication Support System for Older People with Dementia. *IEEE Computer*, 40(5): 35–41.

Amalberti, R. and Valot, C. (1993). From Field Work Analysis to a Cognitive Model and the Design of Support Systems: Assistance to Fighter Pilots. *Proceedings of IEEE Systems Man and Cybernetics Conference*, October 17–20 (Vol. 1, pp. 682–88), Le Touquet, France.

Arnott, J. L. and Alm, N. (2013). Towards the Improvement of Augmentative and Alternative Communication through the Modelling of Conversation. *Computer Speech and Language*, 27(6): 1194–211.

Ashraf, S. and Ricketts, I. W. (2003). Automated Vocabulary Collection to Allow Topical Conversation for Non-speaking People. *Proceedings of HCI International (Universal Access in HCI: Inclusive Design in the Information Society)*, June 22–27, 4 (pp. 181–85). Crete, Greece.

Astell, A., Ellis, M., Bernardi, L., Alm, N., Dye, R., Gowans, G., and Campbell, J. (2010a). Using a Touch Screen Computer to Support Relationships between People with Dementia and Caregivers. *Interacting with Computers*, 22(4): 267–75.

Astell, A., Ellis, M., Alm, N., Dye, R., and Gowans, G. (2010b). Stimulating People with Dementia to Reminisce Using Personal and Generic Photographs. *International Journal of Computers in Healthcare*, 1(2): 177–98.

Balabanović, M., Chu, L. L., and Wolff, G. J. (2000). Storytelling with Digital Photographs. *Proceedings of the ACM SIGCHI Conference on Human Factors in Computing Systems (CHI 2000)*, April 1–6 (pp. 564–71), The Hague, Netherlands.

Ball, L. J., Marvin, C. A., Beukelman, D. R., Lasker, J., and Rupp, D. (1999). Generic Talk Use by Preschool Children. *Augmentative and Alternative Communication*, 15(3): 145–55.

Beattie, G. (1983). *Talk: An Analysis of Speech and Non-Verbal Behaviour in Conversation.* Milton Keynes, UK: Open University Press.

Beukelman, D. R. and Mirenda, P. (2005). *Augmentative and Alternative Communication: Supporting Children and Adults with Complex Communication Needs* (3rd edn). Baltimore, MD: Paul H. Brookes Publishing Company.

Black, R., Reddington, J., Reiter, E., Tintarev, N., and Waller, A. (2010). Using NLG and Sensors to Support Personal Narrative for Children with Complex Communication Needs. *Proceedings of the NAACL HLT 2010 Workshop on Speech and Language Processing for Assistive Technologies* (pp. 1–9), Los Angeles, CA.

Broumley, E. (1994). *TalksBack: The Use of Social Knowledge in an Augmentative Communication System* (Unpublished PhD Thesis). University of Dundee. Dundee, Scotland.

Carpenter, T., McCoy, K., and Pennington, C. (1997). Schema-based Organization of Re-usable Text in AAC: User–Interface Considerations. *Proceedings of the RESNA '97 Annual Conference* (pp. 57–9), Pittsburgh, PA.

Clark, H. H. (1996). *Using Language.* Cambridge, UK: Cambridge University Press.

Clark, H. H. and Schaefer, E. F. (1989). Contributing to Discourse. *Cognitive Science*, 13: 259–94.

Dye, R., Alm, N., Arnott, J. L., Harper, G., and Morrison, A. (1998). A Script-based AAC System for Transactional Interaction. *Natural Language Engineering*, 4(1): 57–71.

Garfinkel, H. (1967). *Studies in Ethnomethodology*. Englewood Cliffs, NJ: Prentice Hall.

Gil, N., Hine, N., Arnott, J. L., Hanson, J., Curry, R., Amaral, T., and Osipovic, D. (2007). Data Visualisation and Data Mining Technology for Supporting Care for Older People. *Proceedings of the ACM SIGACCESS International Conference on Computers and Accessibility (ASSETS 2007)* (pp. 139–46), Tempe, AZ.

Halliday, M. (1985). *An Introduction to Functional Grammar*. London, UK: Edward Arnold.

Harper, G., Dye, R., Alm, N., Arnott, J. L., and Murray, I. R. (1998). A Script-Based Speech Aid for Non-speaking People. *Proceedings of the Institute of Acoustics*, 20(6): 289–95.

Hedvall, P. O. and Rydeman, B. (2010). An Activity Systemic Approach to Augmentative and Alternative Communication. *Augmentative and Alternative Communication*, 26(4): 230–41.

Hedvall, P. O. and Rydeman, B. (2011). A Cultural-Historical Design Approach to Augmentative and Alternative Communication. *Proceedings of the 14th Biennial Conference of the International Society for Augmentative and Alternative Communication (ISAAC 2010)*, Paper O.367, Barcelona, Spain.

Higginbotham, D. J., Moulton, B., Lesher, G., Wilkins, D., and Cornish, J. (2000). Frametalker: Development of a Frame-Based Communication System. *Proceedings of the CSUN Annual International Conference on Technology and Persons with Disabilities*, Los Angeles, CA.

Higginbotham, D. J., Lesher, G. W., Todman, J., File, P., and Wilkins, D. (2002). Utterance-Based Communication: Theory, Research and Design. Short course presented at the *Annual Conference of the Rehabilitation Engineering Society of North America (RESNA 25th International Conference)*, Minneapolis, MN.

Higginbotham, D. J., Kim, K. E., and Scally, C. (2007). The Effect of the Communication Output Method on Augmented Interaction. *Augmentative and Alternative Communication*, 23(2): 140–53.

Hine, N. and Arnott, J. L. (2002). Assistive Social Interaction for Non-speaking People living in the Community. *Proceedings of the 5th International ACM Conference on Assistive Technologies (ASSETS 2002)* (pp. 162–9), Edinburgh, Scotland.

Hine, N., Arnott, J. L., and Smith, D. (2003). Design Issues Encountered in the Development of a Mobile Multimedia Augmentative Communication Service. *Universal Access in the Information Society*, 2(3): 255–64.

Hutchins, E. (1995). *Cognition in the Wild*. Cambridge, MA: MIT Press.

Iwabuchi, M., Alm, N., Andreasen, P., Nakamura, K., and Arnott, J. L. (2001). A Rapid Multi-Lingual Communicator for Non-speaking People and Others. *Proceedings of the IEEE Conference on Systems Man and Cybernetics* (pp. 238–43), Tucson, AZ.

Krivonos, P. and Knapp, M. (1975). Initiating Communication: What Do You Say When You Say Hello? *Central States Speech Journal*, 26(2). Reprinted in B. Morse and L. Phelps (eds), *Interpersonal Communication – A Relational Perspective*. Minneapolis, MN: Burgess Publishing Company.

Laver, J. (1981). Linguistic Routines and Politeness in Greeting and Parting. In F. Coulmas (ed.), *Conversational Routine – Explorations in Standardized Communication Situations and Pre-patterned Speech*. The Hague, Netherlands: Mouton.

Levinson, S. (1983). *Pragmatics*. Cambridge, UK: Cambridge University Press.

Luo, F., Higginbotham, D. J., and Lesher, G. (2007). AAC Webcrawler: Enhanced Augmentative Communication. *Proceedings of the CSUN Annual International Conference on Technology and Persons with Disabilities*, Los Angeles, CA.

Minsky, M. (1975). A Framework for Representing Knowledge. In P. Winston (ed.), *The Psychology of Computer Vision*. New York, NY: McGraw-Hill.

Newell, A. F. (1995). Extra-ordinary Human-Computer Operation. In A. D. N. Edwards (ed.), *Extraordinary Human-Computer Interactions*. London, UK: Cambridge University Press.

O'Mara, D. and Waller, A. (2003). What do you get when you cross a Communication Aid with a Riddle? *The Psychologist*, 16(2): 78–80.

Polkinghorne, D. E. (1995). Narrative Configuration in Qualitative Analysis. In J. A. Hatch and R. Wisniewski (eds), *Life History and Narrative* (pp. 5–24). London, UK: Routledge.

Quasthoff, U. M. and Nikolaus, K. (1982). What Makes a Good Story? Towards the Production of Conversational Narratives, In A. Flammer and W. Kintsch (eds), *Discourse Processing*. Oxford, UK: North-Holland Publishing Co.

Reiter, E., Turner, R., Alm, N., Black, R., Dempster, M., and Waller, A. (2009). Using NLG to Help Language-Impaired Users Tell Stories and Participate in Social Dialogues. *Proceedings of the 12th European Workshop on Natural Language Generation* (Association for Computational Linguistics) (pp. 1–8), Athens, Greece.

Sacks, H., Schegloff, E. A., and Jefferson, G. (1974). A Simplest Systematics for the Organization of Turn-taking for Conversation. *Language*, 50(4): 696–735.

Schank, R. and Abelson, R. P. (1977). *Scripts, Plans, Goals and Understanding: An Inquiry into Human Knowledge Structures*. New York, NY: Erlbaum.

Schegloff, E. A. and Sacks, H. (1973). Opening Up Closings. *Semiotica*, (8)4: 289–327. Abridged version in R. Turner (ed.), *Ethnomethodology* (pp. 233–64). Harmondsworth, UK: Penguin.

Shore, Rima (1997). *Rethinking the Brain: New Insights into Early Development*. New York, NY: Families and Work Institute.

Sienkiewicz-Mercer, R. and Kaplan, S. B. (1989). *I Raise My Eyes To Say Yes*. New York, NY: Houghton Mifflin.

Steele, R. (2004). Benefits of Advanced AAC Technology Uses to Adults with Acquired Aphasia. *AAC Perspectives (ASHA SID-12)*, 13(4): 3–7.

Steele, R., Weinrich, M., Wertz, R., Carlson, G., and Kleczewska, M. (1989). Computer-based Visual Communication in Aphasia. *Neuropsychologia*, 27(4): 409–26.

Todman, J. and Alm, N. (2003). Modelling Conversational Pragmatics in Communication Aids. *Journal of Pragmatics*, 35(4): 523–38.

Todman, J., Alm, N., Higginbotham, J., and File, P. (2008). Whole Utterance Approaches in AAC. *Augmentative and Alternative Communication*, 24(3): 235–54.

Vanderheyden, P. B. (1995). An Augmentative Communication Interface based on Conversational Schemata. *Proceedings of the IJCAI '95 Workshop on Developing AI Applications for Disabled People* (pp. 203–12), Montreal, Canada.

Waller, A. (2006). Communication Access to Conversational Narrative. *Topics in Language Disorders*, 26(3): 221–39.

Waller, A., Dennis, F., Brodie, J., and Cairns, A. Y. (1998). Evaluating the Use of TalksBack, a Predictive Communication Device for Non-fluent Adults with Aphasia. *International Journal of Language and Communication Disorders*, 33(1): 45–70.

Waller, A., Black, R., O'Mara, D. A., Pain, H., Ritchie, G., and Manurung, R. (2009). Evaluating the STANDUP Pun Generating Software with Children with Cerebral Palsy. *ACM Transactions on Accessible Computing*, 1(3): Article 16.

Wang, Y. (2005). *A Linguistic Framework for Technically Augmented Conversational Interaction*. (Unpublished PhD Thesis). University of Dundee, Scotland, UK.

Wisenburn, B. and Higginbotham, D. J. (2008). An AAC Application Using Speaking Partner Speech Recognition to Automatically Produce Contextually Relevant Utterances: Objective Results. *Augmentative and Alternative Communication*, 24(2): 100–09.

Wisenburn, B. and Higginbotham, D. J. (2009). Participant Evaluations of Rate and Communication Efficacy of an AAC Application Using Natural Language Processing. *Augmentative and Alternative Communication*, 25(2): 78–89.

Wittgenstein, L. (1953). *Philosophical Investigations*. Oxford, UK: Basil Blackwell.

Wray, A. (2001). *Formulaic Language and the Lexicon*. London, UK: Cambridge University Press.

Yngve, V. (1970). On Getting a Word in Edgewise. *Papers from the Sixth Regional Meeting of the Chicago Linguistic Society*, 6: 567–78.

8

ASSISTIVE TECHNOLOGY FOR SUPPORTING LEARNING NUMERACY

Pekka Räsänen, Tanja Käser, Anna Wilson, Michael von Aster, Oleksandr Maslov, and Ugné Maslova

Calculation depends on the majority of the abilities within the domain of general intelligence (Blair *et al.*, 2005). Most major theories of intelligence include numeracy or quantitative thinking as one aspect of general cognitive skills (Kaufman *et al.*, 2013). In Chapter 1 of this volume, O'Neill and Gillespie described an example of the cognitively complex social practice of sharing a cup of tea. This activity includes actions like buying tea, measuring the amount of water needed and using a machine to boil it, telephoning a friend's number, and inviting him or her for a visit to a certain address at a certain time. An interesting aspect of this list of actions is that all the activities require using measurement systems or numbers. In fact, numbers and numerical cognition are embedded in our current society. Learning is a cognitively demanding activity and learning or relearning numeracy is particularly demanding. That is why numeracy is one of the key targets of basic education; and may explain the relative scarcity of attempts to rehabilitate mathematical cognition.

Because of the high cognitive demands of quantitative thinking, it is no surprise that humans have developed assistive tools for keeping count, doing calculations, and visualizing numerical, geometrical, and algebraic relations. In addition to tools that are used to assist with calculations, from pebbles (calculus) to calculators (Bogoshi *et al.*, 1987), researchers and educators have invented mechanical machines to assist in learning numeracy. The first patent on an educational device of teaching arithmetic was granted as early as 1897 (Altman, 1897), but it has only been with the recent computer technology and e-learning boom that society has developed a myriad of applications for training basic numerical skills using the Internet, computers, tablets, and mobile phones.

The investigation of technological supports for dyscalculia due to brain injury or degeneration has received relatively little research attention. This is an ironic neglect, as the availability of pocket calculators from 1970 marks the beginning of the information age, an age that has delivered the technology used to support cognition in other areas. A pocket calculator has, to our knowledge, been trialed in one single case of dyscalculia after brain injury (Martins *et al.*, 1999), though their use is often recommended in specific learning disability (e.g. Thompson and Sproule, 2005).

Approaches for adapting mathematical learning tasks will be presented here. These illustrate the possibilities for tasks and materials that could be used in the near future as rehabilitation materials for adults with acquired acalculia (e.g. mathematical disabilities from acquired brain injury or degeneration). The important commonality in these examples is that they all apply current neuroscientific and pedagogical understanding of the cognitive processes required to learn different representations of numbers and their relationships when calculating.

From the inception of mechanical teaching machines, feedback for correct responses (Pressey, 1926), and adaptation to individual skill levels are essential elements of CAL systems (Suppoes and Morningstar, 1972). The majority of current learning applications are able to provide different types of feedback about the user's progress within the tasks, and correct or incorrect responses. Feedback can have many aims; of which, supporting cognitive processes of the learner is only one (see Vasilyeva *et al.* (2007) for a taxonomy of feedback types).

Three models of adaptive learning systems

Here we define assistive technology for learning as technology that adapts according to the learner's needs for learning. There are many ways such a system can adapt. We can identify at least three different main models, which can vary according to the learner's interaction during the learning task (Figure 8.1): the tutor model, the learner model, and the content model.

In the tutor model, an application or a device is designed to mimic the activities of an exemplary human tutor or teacher, an ideal teacher (or a therapist). The system provides feedback and assistance to guide the user to pay attention to relevant information or to use a particular solution strategy to reach the desired solution.

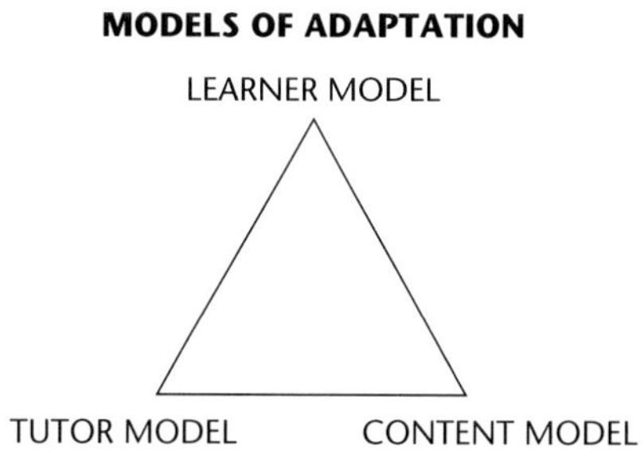

MODELS OF ADAPTATION

LEARNER MODEL

TUTOR MODEL   CONTENT MODEL

FIGURE 8.1   The three models of adaptation for assistive technology for cognition

The tutor model can also provide additional information to the user when the desired progress does not occur. Likewise, the system can, if needed, give feedback to encourage and motivate the learner. New research fields, such as affective computing, allow the integration of emotional aspects into tutor models; for example, incorporating emotional intelligence into intelligent tutoring systems (see e.g. D'Mello *et al.*, 2008; Hussain *et al.*, 2011). Monitoring the user's psychophysiological state may give valid information for the tutor about the user's current levels of motivation, concentration, or even about item-specific emotional reactions to failure or success.

In the learner model, we have a system in which the skills, strategies, or cognitions of the learner are modeled. The system can use response accuracy as its input information, but also solution strategies or response speed. It then uses these to estimate the current level of skills, cognitive profile, or individual rate of learning. This input is used to select the next most suitable item or task to be done, or to modify the feedback needed. Profiling the learner can also be used for selecting different pathways of learning tasks designed to fit to different types of learners. The learner models can also contain diagnostic tasks about the specific types of cognitive or mathematical disorders the user has. This information can be used to build a treatment plan or individualized education plan for the user.

Finally, in the content model, the contents of the task can be organized or ordered in a way that supports learning. Most types of learning content can be ordered according to difficulty, strategic steps or a sequence of categories for which previous information must be mastered before the next content can be studied or learnt properly. Therefore, a learning task based on a content model proceeds according to the learner's development along a predefined order or pathway. A content model can also be a specific numerical activity needed in everyday life. Reduced ability to do mental calculations is a common symptom in various kinds of traumatic brain injuries (TBIs). Mental calculation skills are important, for example, in dealing with money or reading timetables. A content model can consist of tasks for how to do shopping or relearning the clock.

These three adaptive models are not exclusive. Many learning applications or devices use features of all these models. For example, a system can contain a hierarchical, graded or otherwise predefined structure for item selection (content model). Which item will be presented next from this content model can depend on an estimate of the current skill level or cognition of the user (learner model). When not successful, the system can give feedback based on the principles of good pedagogy (tutor model).

Next, we will present three examples of different types of adaptive learning applications, all aiming to support early learning of numeracy. The first, The Number Race, is a simple, adaptive game based on a learner model. The second application is an example of a tutor model; a subtraction task created using an n-dimensionally adaptive Internet application. The last application, Calcularis, is an example of a hybrid learner/content model, which builds individualized pathways of learning using information on the learner's progress within a content model.

Examples of numeracy learning tasks

A learner model: The Number Race game

Wilson and colleagues (Wilson *et al.*, 2006) developed an adaptive computer learning game for children with learning disabilities in mathematics, low numeracy, or in the early stages of learning numeracy in kindergarten. The core concept of The Number Race game is simple. First, the child is required to quickly choose the larger of two quantities presented as groups of objects (e.g. groups of coins or coconuts), written or spoken numerals or, in the highest levels of the game, simple addition or subtraction calculations. In the next step, the child moves their player on a number line board the same number of steps (s)he has selected. The virtual opponent uses the unselected amount of steps, or, if the speed deadline is not reached by the child, the opponent takes the larger number of objects, and therefore steps. The appearance of the game is reminiscent of traditional board games in which one throws a die and advances by that number of steps. The winner is the one who reaches the end of the board first. However, in this game the choice of the two quantities to be compared replaces the dice throw. Furthermore, the difficulty of the items presented is not random, but is constantly adapting based on an artificial intelligence algorithm. This algorithm represents the learner's current skill level ("knowledge space") in three dimensions, and is programmed to ensure an average accuracy of 75 percent. The three dimensions of the model are the ratio of the quantities presented, the time allowed to respond, and the conceptual complexity of the format in which the quantities are presented.

Both the ratio and the speed dimensions in this adaptive algorithm can be seen as an example of a learner model. The ratio of the two quantities to be compared (bigger n/smaller n) has been found to be an important feature in a magnitude comparison process (Feigenson *et al.*, 2004). The larger the ratio, the easier the task is to solve. In practice, this means that a comparison of five versus two objects is easier than seven versus four objects, because the relative difference between the objects to be compared is larger. The cognitive capacity responsible for this selection process has been called the approximate number system (ANS), and is thought to be a specific capacity for perceiving and operating on magnitude. In longitudinal studies, kindergarteners' performance on tasks that draw on the ANS has been found to be highly predictive of numeracy learning in later school years (Mazzocco *et al.*, 2011). It has also been found that children with severe difficulties in learning mathematics need to have a larger ratio to be successful in selecting the larger of two groups of objects (Libertus *et al.*, 2011). However, we also know that the ANS is malleable (DeWind and Brannon, 2012; Piazza *et al.*, 2013). Therefore, this first adaptive dimension (ratio), can be seen as a learner model in that it represents the current level of the user's ability to discriminate ratio (both non-symbolic, i.e. with groups of objects, and symbolic, i.e. with written and/or spoken numerals), and will tend to present subsequent problems at the borders of the user's current skill level.

The second dimension of the adaptive algorithm, speed, can also be considered part of the same learner model. For symbolic numbers (i.e. written and/or spoken numerals), the influence of the ANS is more commonly seen in response speed, rather than accuracy (Dehaene *et al.*, 1990). The speed dimension of the "knowledge space" model represents the user's likely success in meeting the quantity choice deadline at different speeds, and is used to present choices with a deadline that is challenging to the user. The aim is to ensure that the ANS is strongly taxed, or activated, throughout, in order to boost processing in this brain area. By challenging the player to be fast enough to beat the virtual opponent in the game, the speed dimension also contributes to gamification (Kapp, 2012) of the task, and thus motivation and concentration. At higher levels of the third dimension (conceptual complexity), the user is presented with small addition and subtraction problems, and at this level the speed dimension can be seen as a way to push the player to use perception or memory-based strategies over slower counting-based solutions.

The third dimension of the adaptive system, the conceptual complexity, consists of a stepwise progression from comparing concrete objects (e.g. groups of coins or coconuts), to Arabic numbers, and then to simple addition and subtraction problems (with sums under 10). This last dimension can be considered to be a typical content model in which the content of the items has been ordered according to a predefined model of complexity or typical order of learning. In other words, it is a minimalistic school curriculum within the task.

Overall, The Number Race adaptive game is best seen as an example of a learner model. The key function of the adaptive algorithm, and its representation of the child's "knowledge space," is to push the boundaries of the child's knowledge and skill (speed, strategy) of basic number concepts. By doing this, the child is always kept in Vygotsky's "zone of proximal development" where the most efficient learning should occur (Vygotsky, 1978).

A tutor model: learning subtraction

Neure (NEUropsychological Rehabilitation; www.neure.fi) is a web-experimentation system. It is similar to many computer applications built to present stimuli in psychological experiments, except that it runs on java in an Internet browser window. It is mainly used for presenting assessment and intervention tasks for children with learning disabilities. It also contains algorithms to make any task adaptive. The adaptive model implemented is n-dimensional, meaning that any task can be theoretically made to adapt, using any number of dimensions (for technical details see Maslova, 2010).

Building a task with an adaptive logic using the Neure system is simple. The tasks are made of "flash cards" containing auditory or visual stimuli. A user's action or a timer can trigger new contents to be presented, allowing multiple steps within one card. Any interaction of the user with a card can be recorded and classified as a correct or an incorrect answer. To make a task adaptive, the designer has to define dimensions (e.g. difficulty, complexity, and so on). Each card is given values for all these dimensions. This means that each card is positioned in an n-dimensional space (where n is the number of dimensions defined). The user is positioned in this same space. Answering a card then moves the user in each dimension in this space based on predefined values; for example, a correct answer in one direction, and an incorrect answer in the opposite direction. The user's current position is used as an estimate of his/her current level of skills. Each new card is a test of whether that skill has developed or not. As additional features, the system contains randomization options and an option to use item response theory (IRT) values as one dimension (to allow the development of three-parametric assessment tasks with additional rules).

Proof-of-concept experiment

To test these algorithms, we built an experimental task to train subtraction skills with a simple three-dimensional adaptive model. Two of the dimensions described the difficulty of the subtraction task. To keep the model simple, we took the minuend and the difference to be the values of these two dimensions (i.e. if $X - Y = Z$, the dimension values were X and Z). The third and most important dimension was a tutor model divided into three ordered categories: teaching the conceptual understanding of subtraction; teaching subtraction strategies; and training automatization of the subtraction tasks. The tutor model was implemented into seven levels with different types of visualizations and feedback (Figure 8.2). The same subtraction tasks between 2–1 and 18–9 were included in all levels. The tutor model was used to teach more advanced solution strategies to the same calculations in a step-by-step way.

The user starts from the easiest item (which according to the three-dimensional model was $2 - 1 = \underline{}$), presented with a concrete number line visualization to help

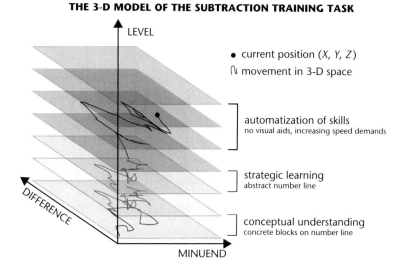

THE 3-D MODEL OF THE SUBTRACTION TRAINING TASK

FIGURE 8.2   The three-dimensional adaptive model of the subtraction training task

conceptual understanding. If the user gave a correct answer, the software moved the user to new co-ordinates in the three-dimensional space and a harder task was given (for example, from $2 - 1 = (1)$ to $4 - 2 = (2)$). In the case of an incorrect answer, corrective feedback and a visualization of the calculation were given and the user moved back to easier items.

The aim of this experiment was to produce a simplified model of an "ideal teacher's behavior" in a string of individualized learning sessions. In a typical classroom setting, children practice subtraction by solving subtraction tasks from their schoolbooks. The teacher monitors the whole classroom and occasionally gives individualized guidance when required. The benefit of the computerized task is that children get immediate feedback on every answer they give, and when they make an error, they get immediate corrective feedback. The adaptive computer task keeps each child at their optimal conceptual level.

We were interested to see if this kind of a model would be beneficial for learning, and thus could be used in the future for e-school books or rehabilitation materials. Four classroom teachers from a local school selected 10 second graders (9-year-olds) for the training on the basis of their showing very low skills in subtraction. According to the curriculum, the children were expected to have mastered these skills in subtraction about a year and a half earlier. The children had short (maximum 15 minutes) daily practice sessions during school breaks. Each child had 12–15 practice sessions in total. The aim of the training task was to support the children in moving gradually from slower counting-based strategies to faster memory retrieval strategies. To achieve this, children were taught first to use 5 and 10 as strategic break-points (that is, to move from "counting all" to shortened counting) and then given repetitive practice for over-learning and to generate strong memory associations between the number combinations.

We measured children's addition and subtraction skills with separate 20-item computerized tasks once before and once after the training. The assessment tasks were presented one at a time on a computer screen, and the children were instructed to respond as fast and accurately as they could. Both accuracy and response speed (in milliseconds) were recorded. The results were clear. Even the poorest performing children at this age were already able to solve addition and subtraction tasks using slow counting-based strategies. Therefore, we did not see improvement in accuracy of performance. However, the response time results showed that there was a significant quantitative and qualitative change in children's calculation skills during the training. There was significant improvement in the median response times both in the non-trained addition ($F = 4{,}373$, $p = 0.043$, Cohen's $d > .5$, indicating a medium level transfer effect) and trained subtraction tasks ($F = 10{,}813$, $p = 0.002$, Cohen's $d > .8$, indicating a large intervention effect).

The graph in Figure 8.3 illustrates the case KA's movements in the space of the two difficulty dimensions at level five (strategic learning) during one training session. He had already mastered the tasks at a conceptual level, but learning to use more advanced calculation strategies seemed to require a lot of practice. The strength of this kind of immediate assistive feedback and adaptive learning task can

Case KA: movements in the task space during one training session (level 5)

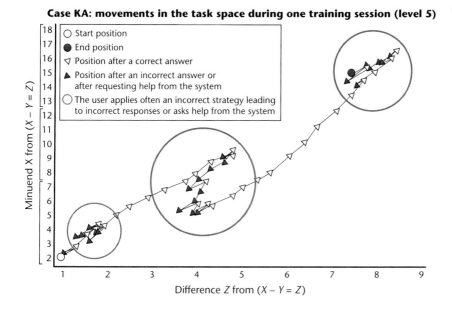

FIGURE 8.3   Performance of the case KA in one training session

be seen from his movements. KA needed several attempts to learn a new strategy suitable for new problem sizes. He was then able to move to larger items (after getting several items correct in a row), but again he seemed to reach a limit of his skills when the items reached a minuend clearly larger above 10 and a difference of close to 8 (e.g. 16–8).

Even though the assistive technology used to learn subtraction was simple, the results were good. Children who had not learnt basic subtraction skills at school within more than a year and a half of instruction, attained fluent solution strategies in less than four hours with individualized, adaptive training that provided immediate feedback and progressive tutoring to more advanced solution strategies. This kind of assistive technology for cognition (ATC) will be at the core of new e-books and e-learning materials, and should be especially useful for children with difficulties in learning. Similar kinds of simple tasks could be used in rehabilitation after TBI or as training materials for adults with dyscalculia.

Calcularis: a combined learner/content model

Calcularis (Käser et al., 2013a) is a computer-based training program for children with difficulties in learning mathematics. To support the learning process, different properties of numbers are encoded through multimodal cues. The learning environment features 3D graphics and interactive components, and thus allows immersion in a playful 3D world. The training program consists of multiple games that are hierarchically structured according to number ranges and can be further

TWO EXAMPLE GAMES FROM THE CALCULARIS

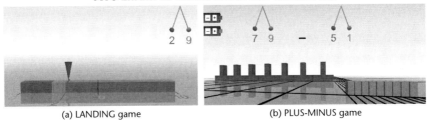

(a) LANDING game   (b) PLUS-MINUS game

FIGURE 8.4   In the LANDING game (a), the position of the displayed number (29) needs to be indicated on the number line. In the PLUS-MINUS game (b), the task displayed needs to be modeled with the blocks of tens and ones

divided into two areas (a content model). The first area (Part A) focuses on different number representations as well as number understanding in general. Transcoding between alternative representations is trained and children learn the three principles of number understanding: cardinality, ordinality, and relativity. The first area is exemplified by the LANDING game illustrated in Figure 8.4(a). In this game, children need to indicate the position of a given number on a number line. To do so, a falling cone has to be steered using a joystick.

The second area (Part B) covers cognitive operations and procedures with numbers. In this area, children train on the concepts and automation of arithmetic operations. In the PLUS-MINUS game (see Figure 8.4(b)), children solve addition and subtraction tasks using blocks of tens and ones to model them. To offer optimal learning conditions, the training program adapts to the knowledge state of a specific child (Käser *et al.*, 2012; Käser *et al.*, 2013b). All children start the training with the same game. After each item, the program estimates the actual knowledge state of the child and displays a new task adjusted to this state.

Learner/content model

In order to adapt the difficulty level and the task selection to the needs of a specific child, the training program needs to represent and estimate the mathematical knowledge of the child. We model this knowledge with a dynamic Bayesian network. This network represents mathematical skills and their dependencies as a directed acyclic graph. Two skills, sA and sB, have a directed connection, if skill sA is a prerequisite for knowing skill sB. Each skill has two states: a learnt state and an unlearnt state. As the skills cannot be observed directly, each skill is associated with certain tasks. The probability that a skill is in the learnt state can then be inferred by evaluating user actions such as correct or wrong answers. At the beginning, all probabilities are set to 0.5, as the system does not know anything about the mathematical knowledge of the children. The probabilities are then updated after each solved task. The probability of a skill therefore changes if a child solves a task that is associated with this skill. Because of the network structure of the model, and the

NUMBER REPRESENTATION SKILLS

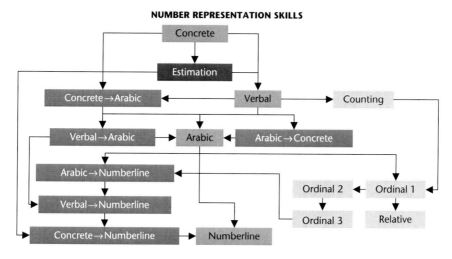

FIGURE 8.5 Number representation skills in the number range 0–100

connections between the skills, the probability of a skill is also influenced when a task associated with one of its precursor or successor skills is solved.

The resulting model consists of 100 different skills, which are assigned to the two parts of the training program. An excerpt of Part A (number representations and number understanding) of the network is displayed in Figure 8.5. Knowledge about number representations include representations of concrete (number as a set of objects), verbal (spoken number), and Arabic numbers (written number) as well as representing the number as a position on a number line (Numberline in Figure 8.5). Likewise, a child needs to acquire the ability to transcode between these different representations. Counting skills connect these representations to principles of ordinality and relativity of numbers. In tasks associated with skill Ordinal 1, the precursor or successor of a number needs to be given. In another task, children are required to add/subtract 10 (or 20 or 30) from a given number (Relative). Skill Ordinal 2 denotes the ability to order numbers according to their magnitude. Finally, children need to guess a number in the range from 0 to 100 (Ordinal 3). In tasks associated with the purple skill, children are required to estimate the quantity of a given set of dots. Skills in Part A are ordered according to the different number ranges 0–10, 0–100, and 0–1,000. Within each number range, the hierarchy follows the four-step developmental model (von Aster and Shalev, 2007). According to this model, transcoding from the linguistic to the Arabic symbolization (Verbal→Arabic) is introduced before training the spatial number line representation (Arabic→Numberline).

Figure 8.6 displays addition skills between 0 and 100, which belong to Part B of the network (cognitive operations and procedures with numbers). Skills in this part can again be sorted into different number ranges. Within a number range, they are ordered according to their difficulties. The difficulty of a task depends on the magnitude of the numbers involved in the task, the complexity of the task, and the

ADDITION SKILL NET IN THE NUMBER RANGE 0–100 WITH EXAMPLE TASKS

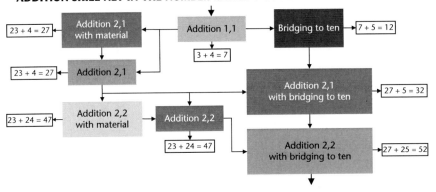

FIGURE 8.6   Addition skill net in the number range 0–100 with example tasks

means allowed to solve the task. Modeling "46 + 33 = 79" with one, ten, and hundred blocks (Support Addition 2,2) is easier than calculating it mentally (Addition 2,2). Furthermore, tasks including a carry such as "46 + 37 = 83" (Addition 2,2 TC) are more complex to solve than tasks not requiring a carry (technical details as well as evaluations of the model can be found in Käser *et al.*, 2012; Käser *et al.*, 2013b).

In order to also be able to adapt to specific problems of a child, the program contains a bug library storing typical error patterns (Gerster, 1982). If a child commits a typical error several times, the controller systematically selects actions for remediation. A typical error pattern is, for example, the switching of digits (25 is written as 52), which is remediated by training transcoding from spoken to written numbers (Verbal→Arabic). Other error patterns occur because of a lack in understanding of the Arabic notation system, i.e. the meaning of the different positions of the digits. The remediation action for these patterns is training of the Arabic notation system (Arabic→Concrete) (a list of all error patterns stored in the bug library can be found in Käser *et al.*, 2013a).

Control

Because of the network structure of the learner/content model, the selection of skills is non-linear. The learning path is adapted for each child. Therefore, each child trains different skills and hence plays different games during training. After each solved task, the control algorithm selects the next task to be solved, based on the probability of the current skill:

- Stay: Continue the training of the current skill.
- Go back: Train a precursor skill.
- Go forward: Train a successor skill.

The decision is based on upper and lower thresholds for the probability of the current skill. The area between the thresholds is considered as being optimal for training. If the probability is higher than the upper threshold, the algorithm selects the "Go forward" option. If the probability is smaller than the lower threshold, the "Go back" option is picked. The thresholds have been chosen heuristically to generate a desired input behavior: About five errors in a row lead to failing a skill, while 10 correct answers are needed to pass a skill.

As a skill can have multiple precursor and successor skills, a set of priority rules is implemented when going back or forward. For the "Go back" option, the algorithm prefers remediation skills; if errors matching patterns of the bug library are detected, the relevant remediation skill is trained. Otherwise, unplayed precursor skills are preferred. The hierarchical skill model assumes that all precursor skills are prerequisites. If the child fails a particular skill, the controller therefore tries to locate the particular precursor skill that caused the problem. For the played precursor skills, the controller assumes that the child already knows them (since they have been played and passed) and hence an unplayed precursor skill is selected. If there is more than one candidate precursor skill left, that with the lowest probability is selected. Therefore, the controller selects the skill for which the child has the lowest proficiency. For the "Go Forward" option, recursion skills are preferred. If a user fails to master skill sA and goes back to sB, sA is set as a recursion skill. After passing sB, the control algorithm will return to sA. If there is more than one candidate successor skill left, the candidate skill with posterior probability closest to 0.5 (maximization of entropy) is selected. This final rule ensures that the gain of knowledge about the child is maximized (the control algorithm and its evaluation are described in detail in Käser et al., 2012; Käser et al., 2013b).

Case study

In order to illustrate the adaptivity of the learning program, the path through the skill net and the training success in subtraction in the number range 0–100 is analyzed for two different children. Both children trained with the program for six weeks. They were required to use the program five times a week in 20-minute sessions. The children and their training characteristics are summarized in Table 8.1.

Figure 8.7 illustrates the path through the network for the two children. The path was quite different for each child. Anne had to go back several times and

TABLE 8.1 Characteristics of the two children

	Sex	Age	Class	Played sessions	Solved tasks	Tasks per session
Anne	female	8;11	3	28	1,272	45.4
Jane	female	9;10	4	33	1,795	54.4

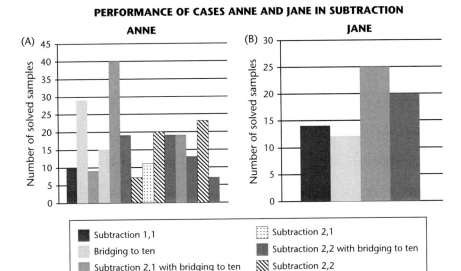

PERFORMANCE OF CASES ANNE AND JANE IN SUBTRACTION

ANNE

JANE

■ Subtraction 1,1

▦ Subtraction 2,1

░ Bridging to ten

▨ Subtraction 2,2 with bridging to ten

▒ Subtraction 2,1 with bridging to ten

⧅ Subtraction 2,2

FIGURE 8.7 Skill sequence and played samples in subtraction in the number range 0–100 from Anne (a) and Jane (b)

consolidate more basic skills, while Jane followed the shortest path through the network. While Anne solved 241 tasks in subtraction between 0 and 100, Jane passed this section after 71 tasks. The external training effects in subtraction from 0 to 100 (measured by a computer-based subtraction test), reveal the same patterns. Before the training, Jane solved 39 tasks of the test correctly, while Anne solved only 10 tasks correctly. After the training, Anne solved 23 tasks correctly and especially improved in subtraction that required carrying. Jane solved 49 tasks correctly after the training. However, she mostly improved in subtraction tasks in the number range 0–1,000.

The effects of the training program have been assessed in a study with 41 children conducted in Switzerland. Participants were divided into a training group that completed 12 weeks of training and a waiting group starting with a 6-week rest period. The results revealed positive training effects in mathematical skills after completion of the training. Children significantly improved their subtraction skills over the course of six weeks training. Children were also able to locate the position of a number on a number line more accurately after training. In the number range 0–10, the deviation from the correct position was reduced by 33 percent after six weeks. Furthermore, prolongation of the training from six to 12 weeks yielded a beneficial effect. After 12 weeks, children also improved significantly in addition, and were able to locate the position of a number on a number line more accurately in higher number ranges (a detailed description and discussion of the evaluation study and the results can be found in Käser, *et al.*, 2013a).

The future of assistive technologies for learning numeracy

The technical revolution in education is bringing adaptive technologies for cognition into homes, workplaces, and classrooms. ATC will challenge the ways in which we have traditionally organized education and learning. Unlike traditional books, e-learning materials can contain various types of assistive systems that adapt according to users' needs, skills, and cognition. ATC enables individualization of learning content and tutoring, and particularly for us to take into account individual differences in cognition and learning. Similar approaches could be used in rehabilitation. However, there is an urgent need for research on suitable models.

An ATC that implements an adaptive learner model can be multimodal. Not only can it contain domain-specific knowledge and processes of numeracy, as in our examples, but it can also include embedded assessment of motivational states (Kickmeier-Rust et al., 2011) and even biofeedback or online measures of brain activity (Galán and Beal, 2012; Mostow et al., 2011). The increasing processing power of computers allows for an increasing number of variables or dimensions to be handled by the adaptive models.

One of the biggest challenges faced in developing assistive technologies for numerical cognition comes from the very nature of numbers and quantities. Numbers are ubiquitous in our world, and magnitude is a basic feature of every perceptual input (Stoianov and Zorzi, 2012). There is always an amount in or of everything. Whether this information about an amount or number is relevant for decision-making or for actions is situation dependent. It is impossible to model all the everyday situations in which basic skills in number and/or calculation are required. Assistive technologies for using numeracy must, therefore, be more or less task specific. We will thus see a rapid growth in assistive technologies for learning numeracy, but not for using numeracy. The development of technologies using natural language processing in the future could provide support for the latter. A person with mathematical disabilities can describe the situational demands and information available, and the system can guide the person through the decision process (Cercone and Naruedomkul, 2013; Pascual-Nieto et al., 2011).

Simple models of this kind of tool are already widely available. While paper-and-pencil algorithms and calculators used to be the main tools to solve calculations when a person was not able do so mentally, these days smartphones connected to Internet databases and computational knowledge engines, such as Wolfram Alpha, can provide answers to verbally spoken numerical tasks. The results are presented in various ways to aid understanding from numbers to graphs. Likewise, complex numerical information can be read with the smartphone cameras from bar or QR codes, and this information can be used directly to pay bills or do shopping, without the need for calculations. These codes can also be attached to numerical information to guide a person to additional information needed to understand the meaning of the numbers in that context.

The ATC applications reviewed above are challenging the traditional ways education and rehabilitation of numerical cognition have been conducted, as may new knowledge on neuroscientific approaches, which can directly affect neural activation during learning (e.g. Cohen Kadosh *et al.* 2010). However, the only certain fact is that what we see now is just the beginning. The results of revolutions are often substantially different from that which their instigators envisaged.

References

Altman, G. G. (1897). *Apparatus for Teaching Arithmetic*. Washington, DC: United States Patent Office; No. 588,371.

Blair, C., Gamson, D., Thorne, S., and Baker, D. (2005). Rising Mean IQ: Cognitive Demand of Mathematics Education for Young Children, Population Exposure to Formal Schooling and the Neurobiology of the Prefrontal Cortex. *Intelligence*, 33(1): 93–106.

Bogoshi, J., Naidoo, K., and Webb, J. (1987). The Oldest Mathematical Artefact. *Mathematical Gazette*, 71(458): 294.

Cercone, N. J. and Naruedomkul, K. (2013). *Computational Approaches to Assistive Technologies for People with Disabilities* (Vol. 253). Amsterdam, Netherlands: IOS Press.

Cohen Kadosh, R., Soskic, S., Iuculano, T., Kanai, R., and Walsh, V. (2010). Modulating Neuronal Activity Produces Specific and Long-lasting Changes in Numerical Competence. *Current Biology*, 20(22): 2016–20.

Dehaene, S., Dupoux, E., and Mehler, J. (1990). Is Numerical Comparison Digital? Analogical and Symbolic Effects in Two-Digit Number Comparison. *Journal of Experimental Psychology: Human Perception and Performance*, 16(3): 626–41.

DeWind, N. K. and Brannon, E. M. (2012). Malleability of the Approximate Number System: Effects of Feedback and Training. *Frontiers in Human Neuroscience*, 6(68): 1–10. Available at: www.ncbi.nlm.nih.gov/pmc/articles/PMC3329901/pdf/fnhum-06-00068.pdf (accessed 26 September 2014).

D'Mello, S., Jackson, T., Craig, S., Morgan, B., Chipman, P., White, H., Person, N., Kort, B., El Kaliouby, R., Picard, R., and Graesser, A. (2008). AutoTutor Detects and Responds to Learners' Affective and Cognitive States. In *Proceedings of the Workshop on Emotional and Cognitive Issues in ITS in Conjunction with the 9th International Conference on Intelligent Tutoring Systems* (pp. 31–43). Available at: www.cs.memphis.edu/%7Esdmello/assets/papers/dmello-affectwkshp-its08.pdf (accessed 26 September 2014).

Feigenson, L., Dehaene, S., and Spelke, E. (2004). Core Systems of number. *Trends in Cognitive Sciences*, 8(7): 307–14.

Galán, F. C. and Beal, C. R. (2012). EEG Estimates of Engagement and Cognitive Workload Predict Math Problem Solving Outcomes. In *User Modeling, Adaptation and Personalization* (pp. 51–62). New York, NY: Springer.

Gerster, H. D. (1982). *Schülerfehler bei Schriftlichen Rechenverfahren*. Freiburg, Germany: Herder.

Hussain, M. S., AlZoubi, O., Calvo, R. A., and D'Mello, S. K. (2011). Affect Detection from Multichannel Physiology During Learning Sessions with AutoTutor. In *Artificial Intelligence in Education* (pp. 131–8). New York, NY: Springer.

Kapp, K. M. (2012). *The Gamification of Learning and Instruction: Game-Based Methods and Strategies for Training and Education*. New York, NY: John Wiley and Sons.

Käser, T., Busetto, A. G., Baschera, G. M., Kohn, J., Kucian, K., Von Aster, M., and Gross, M. (2012). Modelling and Optimizing the Process of Learning Mathematics. *Proceedings of ITS*, 7315 (pp. 389–98). doi: 10.1007/978-3-642-30950-2_50.

Käser, T., Baschera, G. M., Kohn, J., Kucian, K., Richtmann, V., Grond, U., and Von Aster, M. (2013a). Design and Evaluation of The Computer-Based Training Program Calcularis for Enhancing Numerical Cognition. *Frontiers in Psychology*, 4. doi: 10.3389/fpsyg.2013.00489.

Käser, T., Busetto, A. G., Solenthaler, B., Baschera, G. M., Kohn, J., Kucian, K., Von Aster, M., and Gross, M. (2013b). Modelling and Optimizing Mathematics Learning in Children. *International Journal of Artificial Intelligence in Education*, 23: 115–35. doi: 10.1007/s40593-013-0003-7.

Kaufman, J. C., Kaufman, S. B., and Plucker, J. A. (2013). *Contemporary Theories of Intelligence. Oxford Handbook of Cognitive Psychology*. Oxford, UK: Oxford University Press.

Kickmeier-Rust, M. D., Mattheiss, E., Steiner, C., and Albert, D. (2011). A Psycho-pedagogical Framework for Multi-Adaptive Educational Games. *International Journal of Game-Based Learning*, 1(1): 45–58.

Libertus, M. E., Feigenson, L., and Halberda, J. (2011). Preschool Acuity of the Approximate Number System Correlates with School Math Ability. *Developmental Science*, 14(6): 1292–300.

Martins, I. P., Ferreira, J., and Borges, L. (1999). Acquired Procedural Dyscalculia Associated to a Left Parietal Lesion in a Child. *Child Neuropsychology*, 5: 265.

Maslova, U. (2010). *A Multidimensional Adaptive System for Web-based Computer Assisted Learning: A Model and an Implementation*. Tampere, Finland: Tampere University of Technology.

Mazzocco, M. M., Feigenson, L., and Halberda, J. (2011). Impaired Acuity of the Approximate Number System Underlies Mathematical Learning Disability (Dyscalculia). *Child Development*, 82(4): 1224–37.

Mostow, J., Chang, K. M., and Nelson, J. (2011). Toward Exploiting EEG Input in a Reading Tutor. In *Artificial Intelligence in Education* (pp. 230–7). New York, NY: Springer.

Pascual-Nieto, I., Santos, O. C., Perex-Marin, D., and Boticario, J. G. (2011). Extending Computer Assisted Assessment Systems with Natural Language Processing, User Modeling and Recommendations Based on Human Computer Interaction and Data Mining. In *Proceedings of the Twenty-Second International Joint Conference on Artificial Intelligence, Volume Three* (pp. 2519–24). Palo Alto, CA: AAAI Press.

Piazza, M., Pica, P., Izard, V., Spelke, E. S., and Dehaene, S. (2013). Education Enhances the Acuity of the Nonverbal Approximate Number System. *Psychological Science*, 24(6): 1037–43.

Pressey, S. L. (1926). A Simple Apparatus which gives Tests and Scores – and Teaches. *School and Society*, 23 (586): 373–6.

Stoianov, I. and Zorzi, M. (2012). Emergence of A-visual Number Sense in Hierarchical Generative Models. *Nature Neuroscience*, 15(2): 194–6.

Suppoes, P. and Morningstar, M. (1972). *Computer-assisted Instruction at Stanford, 1966–68: Data, Models and Evaluation of the Arithmetic Programs*. New York, NY: Academic Press.

Thompson, T. and Sproule, S. (2005). Calculators for Students with Special Needs. *Teaching Children Mathematics*, 11(7): 391–5.

Vasilyeva, E., Puuronen, S., Pechenizkiy, M., and Räsänen, P. (2007). Feedback Adaptation in Web-Based Learning Systems. *International Journal of Continuing Engineering Education and Life Long Learning*, 17(4): 337–57.

Von Aster, M. G. and Shalev, R. S. (2007). Number Development and Developmental Dyscalculia. *Developmental Medicine and Child Neurology*, 49(11): 868–73.

Vygotsky, L. S. (1978). *Mind in Society: The Development of Higher Psychological Processes*. Cambridge, MA: Harvard University Press.

Wilson, A. J., Dehaene, S., Pinel, P., Revkin, S. K., Cohen, L., and Cohen, D. (2006). Principles Underlying the Design of "The Number Race," an Adaptive Computer Game for remediation of Dyscalculia. *Behavioral and Brain Functions*, 2(1): 19.

9

ASSISTIVE TECHNOLOGY FOR PSYCHOMOTOR FUNCTIONING AND SEQUENCING COMPLEX MOVEMENTS

Jennifer Boger and Alex Mihailidis

Being able to engage in work, leisure, and self-care activities is a key component of identity and wellbeing. Impaired psychomotor functioning and impaired movement sequencing can limit a person's ability to interact with their environment, placing constraints on what activities they are able to do. This chapter presents intelligent assistive technologies that are intended to augment or, in some cases, rehabilitate psychomotor functioning to enable people with impairments to participate more fully in their lives. The chapter begins by introducing psychomotor functioning and how a cognitive impairment can impact a person's ability to complete activities, followed by an overview of zero-effort intelligent assistive technologies for cognition and why this class of technology is well suited to supporting psychomotor functioning. Intelligent powered wheelchairs, computer-guided support for people with dementia, and robot-guided post-stroke rehabilitation are presented as examples of application areas, along with examples of research being done in each. The chapter concludes with some general thoughts about assistive technology for cognition and speculation regarding challenges that lie ahead.

What is psychomotor functioning?

Being able to participate in the world is central to maintaining one's health, independence, and overall sense of wellbeing. Defined by the field of occupational therapy, *occupation* refers to the "active process of living: from the beginning to the end of life. Occupations are all the active processes of looking after ourselves and others, enjoying life, and being socially and economically productive over the lifespan and in various contexts" (Townsend, 1997: 19). In this context, occupation refers to all the tasks that people do, ranging from routine everyday chores to significant once-in-a-lifetime achievements. Thus, occupations are a significant part of one's identity; who we are is a reflection of what we have done, are able and choose to do, and hope to do in the future (Dickie, 2009).

Psychomotor functioning refers to the cognitive processes associated with motor activity, such as hand and eye coordination or gait (World Health Organization, 2002; Üstün *et al.*, 2003). Psychomotor functioning encompasses one's ability to process sensory information cognitively and engage in appropriate muscle activity to produce movements with correct direction, amplitude, and timing of movement, to achieve a desired outcome (Sathian *et al.*, 2011). In healthy individuals, psychomotor abilities are learned over the course of a lifetime and improve with practice. Psychomotor acts are controlled by explicit memory for the sequence or procedural memory and the more a psychomotor ability is practiced, the less conscious cognitive effort is required (Proctor and Dutta, 1995). Playing a musical instrument requires focused attention, mediation of movement by explicit memory, and many hours of practice to learn the cognitive mappings corresponding to the intended interactions with the instrument. The greater a musician's ability with an instrument, the more cognitively effortless playing becomes. Psychomotor function allows transfer of skills to other activities; a talented musician can learn new styles of music or other instruments much more readily than can a novice.

Successful completion of an activity requires that a person is able to define what they would like to achieve through the activity, create a plan about how to reach their goal, execute the steps required to complete the activity (which often has a sequence that must be completed in the correct order), and react to unanticipated deviations. Healthy psychomotor functioning entails not simply being able to sequence and execute steps in an activity, but also being able to handle when an activity does not proceed as expected by recognizing that a deviation has occurred then either changing the goal or identifying and implementing an alternate pathway of steps to attain the original goal. This plasticity enables a walking person to keep his balance when he is bumped into and an experienced musician to improvise in style and tempo to play with other musicians.

Difficulties in psychomotor functioning follow many types of injury or illness of the brain. Prognosis for psychomotor recovery depends on factors such as pathology, volume and region of affected brain tissue, age, and psychomotor development at the time of injury. Impairments caused by a traumatic brain injury or stroke are worst just after the adverse event as they are an acute injury and can often improve because of brain plasticity. Other conditions, such as most of the dementias, are characterized by progressively worsening over time (World Health Organization, 2012). Often, a person with compromised psychomotor abilities will require assistance with daily tasks. The amount and type of assistance depends on functional abilities, health, and personal preferences. Whether assistance is provided by a human or by technology, it must be appropriately matched to each individual's needs, abilities, and preferences for it to be accepted and effective (Scherer *et al.*, 2005; Schulz *et al.*, 2012).

Zero-effort intelligent technology for cognition

Increasingly powerful computer-based technologies and systems have resulted in significant advancements in the field of applied *artificial intelligence (AI)*. AI refers to the ability of a computer-based agent (i.e. processor or system) to apply some form of logic to its understanding of the world to make rational decisions. An AI agent uses a set of rules to select an optimal course of action based on sensor-derived knowledge of the state of the world (Russell and Norvig, 2010).

Abstractly, AI agents can be thought of as having three modules: sensing, decision making, and action implementation (Figure 9.1). Sensing is how an AI agent captures what is going on in the world. This information is passed along to the decision-making module, which applies a computational model to determine what is happening and what is the best course of action to take (including taking no action). The action implementation module executes the action selected by the decision-making module. Hence, an AI agent operates by continuously capturing data, making a decision about what action to take based on this data, then doing the action. There are many AI techniques available, covering a broad range of complexity and granularity. The technique (or techniques) selected for each module depends on the application. Different techniques can be used by each module and not all modules need to use an AI-based technique for the overall device or system to have AI capabilities. For example, a hypothetical system might use AI computer vision techniques to recognize and track a specific object autonomously (e.g. the location of a person's keys) using a stream of video data. This data could be passed to a decision-making module that applies its own AI techniques to analyze the incoming information continuously and makes a decision regarding what action to take (e.g. every second, the device decides whether or not to play a message telling the person where their keys are). The decision is passed to the action implementation module, which could consist of a simple look-up table that maps each decision to a pre-recorded prompt. Depending on the application, these modules can be expanded to include sub-systems or combined into a single system; however,

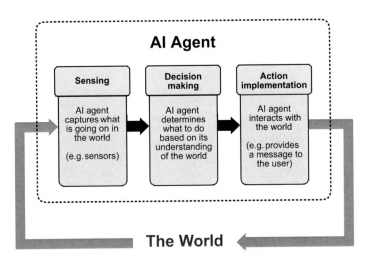

FIGURE 9.1 Conceptualization of the modules that make up an AI agent

regardless of the technical operation, the important aspect of an AI-based system is that it is able to perform some level of autonomous decision making.

The application of AI to assistive technologies for cognition results in devices and systems that are able to make decisions with little or no explicit input from the people using them. These *intelligent technologies for cognition* (ITCs) have tremendous potential for supporting psychomotor functioning as they are able to complement and support compromised cognitive functions by assisting with decision making. Moreover, ITCs can be designed to learn about the preferences and needs of the people using them, enabling ITCs to provide customized support that matches abilities, and dynamically change over time. ITCs can support psychomotor functioning by helping to teach people new abilities, relearn affected abilities or augment abilities that have been compromised.

A fundamental goal of technology design is ease of use. Technologies that require little or no effort to operate are considered to be *zero-effort technologies* (Mihailidis *et al.*, 2011). It is important to clarify that a zero-effort technology may require the person using it to exert mental or physical effort; however, this effort is intentionally and constructively directed toward the activity or task rather than toward the operation of the technology (Mihailidis *et al.*, 2011). For example, relearning a psychomotor task following an illness often requires tremendous and persistent mental and physical effort. An ITC for task relearning could continually encourage the user to perform to the fullest extent of his or her abilities, thereby expanding his or her skills. Ideally, an ITC is able to learn about the person using it, autonomously estimate preferences and what level of effort (cognitive, physical, or otherwise) is reasonable to expect, and adapt to the user as his or her preferences or abilities change. Being able to adjust parameters dynamically to match the abilities and goals of an individual, without the user (or their caregiver or clinician) having to change the device or system settings, is of particular relevance to supporting cognitive impairments as people from these populations may not be able to operate a device reliably or intentionally and their caregivers are often unable to do so on the care recipient's behalf.

Developing an ITC is a complex endeavor that requires the close collaboration of a multidiscipline team. To ensure that technologies can be used to support the user's task-directed efforts, ITCs should involve representative end-users throughout the design process to ensure the final product meets their needs (Shah *et al.*, 2009). In addition to increased adoption rates, involving representative end-users increases safety and reduces user errors (Galway *et al.*, 2013). Unfortunately, involving representative end-users is not always feasible because of time, budget, and limited access to the population of interest. Part of the challenge of developing effective ITCs is to employ methods (that may or may not include representative end-users) to maximize the potential applicability of the proposed solutions. This includes evaluating the effectiveness of an ITC and comparing its performance to other solutions so that successful strategies may be identified and developed further. The knowledge gained through a development effort should be disseminated appropriately, including moving the ITC toward a commercially available product if possible.

The remainder of this chapter presents examples to illustrate how a few of the commonly occurring impairments in different populations and contexts can be supported by zero-effort ITCs. These examples are by no means exhaustive; rather, they are intended to give the reader a feel for the capabilities and versatility of high-tech devices and systems for supporting psychomotor functioning.

Mobility assistance by intelligent powered wheelchairs

Mobility enables us to get from place to place. Being mobile has many benefits, including: achievement of personal goals such as seeing desired people and places, positive psychological effects of being able to take up opportunities, physiological wellbeing from getting exercise, involvement in the community and social networks, and the reassurance of being able to get to another place when needed or chosen (Metz, 2000). Mobility enables access to occupations that are key to a person's independence, wellbeing, and quality of life (Spinney et al., 2009; Bourret et al., 2002).

In conditions where ambulation is significantly impaired, typically a person will use a wheelchair to enable mobility. Power-assisted wheelchairs are useful where a lack of strength or endurance prevents operation of a manual wheelchair. Similarly, people with hemiplegia (i.e. paralysis of one side of the body) and cerebral palsy often require powered wheelchairs to achieve mobility. However, driving a powered wheelchair requires motor skills, good planning, judgment, and reaction time. The driver must ensure that the path he or she is taking is clear of potential obstacles and hazards, must be able to anticipate and compensate for unexpected situations (e.g. a person stepping in front of the chair), and must be able to react in time to avoid a collision. Often, the changes in cognition that accompany conditions such as dementia, stroke, traumatic brain injury, and cerebral palsy result in insufficient cognitive and/or psychomotor skills to operate a powered wheelchair safely. Thus while people with cognitive impairments may require a wheelchair for mobility, safety concerns for the wheelchair driver and the surrounding people and environment frequently prohibit access to powered wheelchairs (Mortenson et al., 2006). If they cannot propel themselves manually, the cognitively impaired person is reliant on caregivers to get to desired destinations or simply to explore his or her environment. This can have the negative consequences of reduced mobility, loss of independence, increased caregiver burden, and decreased feelings of wellbeing.

A powered wheelchair with AI may be able to complement the driver's cognitive abilities, ensuring safe powered wheelchair operation. This could provide people with cognitive impairments access to powered mobility, thus enhancing quality of life and wellbeing (Simpson et al., 2008). Since the 1980s there have been several intelligent wheelchairs developed for a variety of populations, both with and without cognitive impairments. Simpson (2005) provides a comprehensive literature review of intelligent wheelchairs, which we here update with some of the systems that have been developed since the completion of the review.

Boucher *et al.* (2013) developed an intelligent powered wheelchair that can perform accurate, autonomous maneuvering in constrained spaces. In addition to normal driving capabilities, the chair has three tasks it could perform autonomously: wall following (i.e. the chair follows a wall at a set distance away), parking (i.e. the chair approaches and stops at environmental features, such as a table), and door frame traversal, which is a challenging maneuver for both human and autonomous wheelchair because of the tight fit. The chair can be driven using a conventional joystick method, but also has speech recognition capabilities that allow the driver to control the chair through vocal commands. The sensing module of the wheelchair detects free/occupied space around the chair (using three planar laser rangefinders) and keeps track of characteristics such as the chair's speed and inertia. The decision-making module of the chair uses this information to execute the desired task selected by the user, avoid collisions, and navigate around obstacles. The modular design of the chair means that its capabilities can be expanded relatively easily by adding more modules as they are developed. For instance, future work includes the addition of mapping to help navigate in larger, unknown environments. The chair achieved good results with a test group of healthy and representative users who had physical disabilities. Areas identified for future improvement include fixing technical difficulties with the lasers and misinterpreted speech commands by the speech recognition module. Importantly, Boucher *et al.* (2013) created the Robotic Wheelchair Skills Test (RWST). Based on the Wheelchair Skills Test, which was developed and validated by Kirby *et al.* (2004), the RWST examines 15 wheelchair maneuvers that could benefit from AI-guided or AI-assisted control. The RWST provides a methodology for intelligent powered wheelchair developers to quantify and compare the performance of different designs, enabling critical performance appraisal and support of intelligent powered wheelchair development in general by helping to identify the approaches that are more successful. While the wheelchair discussed above has only been tested with cognitively-able individuals, it is not difficult to envision how the functionality and interface could be adapted to complement people with cognitive impairments.

Sonar, lasers, and infra-red rangefinders have been used as the sensors for many autonomous wheelchair designs. However, these designs often run into problems with reflective surfaces, noise from ambient sources (e.g. sunlight), conflicting readings when there are multiple chairs using the same type of sensor, and a limited ability to detect objects at heights (e.g. the edge of a table) (Simpson, 2005). One way to overcome these problems is to use a stereovision-based system (i.e. the use of multiple cameras to capture a 3-D image). While the processing demands of stereovision are higher than other sensors, it does have the advantages of fewer problems with noise and the ability to perform multiple functions, such as object recognition as well as depth perception. One such vision-based wheelchair has been developed to avoid collisions as well as to provide the driver with verbal prompts to assist him or her in navigating around obstacles and get to a desired target (e.g. "Try turning left") (How *et al.*, 2013; Viswanathan *et al.*, 2012; Viswanathan *et al.*, 2011). In addition, the vision capabilities of the chair can be combined with AI mapping techniques, enabling the wheelchair to autonomously map a new environment and perform localization and navigation tasks in it. The wheelchair performed well in pilot tests with older adults with dementia, significantly decreasing participants' collision rates and driving distances during driving tasks in a controlled setting. Feedback from the users about perceived usability varied considerably and was correlated with the level of dementia and the chair's accuracy. Namely, participants who were more cognitively aware understood that the chair was providing assisted driving, were more accepting of the guidance it offered and had a greater tolerance for incorrect prompts.

Many intelligent wheelchairs provide anti-collision capabilities or autonomously perform certain tasks (e.g. wall following) and navigation objectives (e.g. driving to a destination). This style of control is not ideal for many users, as it can create frustration and confusion when the chair "takes over" (Urdiales *et al.*, 2011; Viswanathan *et al.*, 2011). Moreover, having the chair do all the skilled driving does not encourage the driver to practice using his or her residual skills. Urdiales *et al.* (2011) developed a *shared control algorithm* that enabled control of the wheelchair to be shared simultaneously between a computerized agent and the human driver. The algorithm is able to learn about the driver's abilities and to adjust the amount of autonomous control of the wheelchair accordingly, with more of an emphasis on human control for more adept drivers and more robotic control (e.g. autonomous anti-collision and navigation) for drivers with greater cognitive or physical impairments. The goal of the shared control paradigm is to encourage the driver to stay as actively involved in driving as possible without jeopardizing safety. Trials with 18 participants with mixed levels of cognition and physical abilities resulted in every participant reaching their intended destination, although some found the control paradigm to be more useful than did others. The participants who had the most trouble with the chair were the ones with high cognitive functioning and low physical abilities. The authors speculate that this was because these drivers recognized the chair was augmenting control and actively "fought" the chair if it did not do exactly what they wished. While the chair enabled the drivers to reach their goal, more work needs to be done into understanding how to mesh autonomous control with users' preferences and abilities.

As can be seen through the above examples, it is extremely difficult for developers to anticipate how their wheelchair design will react to different types of drivers. In an effort to mitigate this problem, Peula *et al.* (2012) have been working to create a case-based reasoning emulator that simulates different types of wheelchair drivers. The emulator is trained with data from real-world drivers with different abilities completing maneuvers of interest (e.g. turning corners, navigating doorways, and so on). Preliminary tests with simple maneuvers showed good agreement between simulated driving paths using the emulator and paths from real users. The authors intend to expand the work to more complex scenarios with the hope of creating a tool that provides realistic simulations that developers could use to test proposed algorithms so that the resulting systems are more robust and suitable to users' needs.

Computerized guidance of activities of daily living for people living with dementia

Dementia is an umbrella term that encompasses conditions where a person's cognitive abilities are affected enough to cause difficulties with daily functioning (Merriam-Webster Medical Dictionary, 2014). Alzheimer's Disease and other dementias impact several areas of cognition, including memory, planning, abstract thinking, language, and motor skills, which usually translate into a significant impairment in a person's psychomotor abilities (Kluger *et al.*, 1997). As the symptoms that accompany dementia worsen, changes in memory and psychomotor functioning hinder a person's ability to complete the occupations that are necessary to maintain health, independence, and a sense of wellbeing. Research suggests that, in addition to being enjoyable, staying engaged in occupations and maintaining a good sense of wellbeing may slow cognitive decline, including with dementias such as Alzheimer's Disease (Daviglus *et al.*, 2010). While participating in occupations is beneficial, many people with dementia cannot do so without assistance as they have trouble remembering the sequence of steps in the task or how to complete the steps themselves. The conventional solution is to have a formal (i.e. paid) or informal (e.g. family or friend) caregiver supervise the person with dementia as they complete a task to remind him or her of steps he or she misses or simply complete the task outright. This places tremendous burden on caregivers and can cause feelings of dependence, inadequacy, and low self-esteem for the care recipient (Clyburn *et al.*, 2000; Torti *et al.*, 2004). It has been shown that "hours per day spent caring" is a major factor of caregiver burden (Bruvik *et al.*, 2013). Additionally, most people with dementia want to remain actively involved in their own lives for as long as possible (Fetherstonhaugh *et al.*, 2013). About 64 percent of people with Alzheimer's Disease, the most common form of dementia, are living at home, with 53 percent living with a caregiver and the other 11 percent living alone (Craig *et al.*, 2005). During the early stages of dementia, a person has only a mild cognitive impairment (MCI) and is usually capable of living alone. However, increasing cognitive impairments result in greater difficulties with sequencing movements involved in activities of daily living (e.g. toileting, bathing, and meal preparation), which are necessary for healthy independent living.

There have been several ITCs created with the goal of supporting people with dementia. One example is the mobile phone-based video streaming (MPVS) system, designed to provide users with mild Alzheimer's Disease with video reminders of how to complete tasks (Galway *et al.*, 2013; O'Neill *et al.*, 2011). Reminders are recorded and scheduled by a caregiver and played back to the user with dementia over a mobile phone platform, which has a single button that the person with dementia pushes to acknowledge the message. The infrastructure allows for the caregiver to manage reminders remotely from the person with dementia, fostering peace of mind and independence for both. MPVS was created with input from 72 participants (i.e. people with dementia and their caregivers) and results from use with test groups showed a high acceptance rate. While the reminders are currently scheduled by a caregiver, it is easy to see how a device such as this could be integrated into a more autonomous smart-home in the future. Notably, the researchers used their experiences and data from developing the MPVS system to analyze carefully the device's performance, identify factors that influenced technology uptake, and create a model that can be used to predict whether a specific person with dementia/caregiver dyad will be likely adaptors of the technology (O'Neill *et al.*, 2014). While the model is currently specific to the MPVS system, it demonstrates how, given more data, a more complex predictive model might be created that could be tremendously useful in matching people to technologies that they would find helpful. The researchers also used the MPVS project to illustrate a proposed design framework that developers can use to promote stakeholder involvement and user-centered design (Galway *et al.*, 2013).

COACH is another example of ITC designed to assist people with dementia to complete activities of daily living. COACH operates by tracking a person with dementia as they complete an activity and providing audio/video cues to help guide the person through missed or incorrectly completed steps in the activity (Mihailidis *et al.*, 2008b). Secondary goals of COACH are to preserve cognitive skills by encouraging people with dementia to complete the task with minimal assistance (i.e. the "use it or lose it" principle) and to foster feelings of independence, dignity, and autonomy. COACH is able to learn about each user over time, allowing COACH to get a sense of how much assistance he or she requires on any given day and keep track of his or her overall (long-term) abilities. This enables COACH to match prompts to a person's abilities, giving succinct prompts to someone functioning at a higher cognitive level and more detailed cues to someone who requires more assistance. Importantly, COACH uses computer vision that can perform markerless tracking, which means that the person does not have to wear anything or push a button for COACH to work. Engineers, computer scientists, rehabilitation scientists, healthcare professionals, informal caregivers, and people with dementia have worked as a transdisciplinary team on five iterations of COACH, with each version building on results from trials with the previous prototype (Boger *et al.*, 2006; Czarnuch *et al.*, 2013; Hoey *et al.*, 2010; Mihailidis *et al.*, 2008a; Mihailidis *et al.*, 2008b; Mihailidis *et al.*, 2001). Each version has been tested in a long-term care environment with participants who have moderate-to-severe dementia and has shown promising results. The majority of participants are able to complete more steps in the handwashing task without help from a caregiver and some are able to wash their hands without any assistance from a caregiver. Moreover, most participants accept the technology, as demonstrated by their willingness to comply with prompts and, in some cases, by responding with amicable conversation to verbal prompts. In the latest trials, COACH ran unsupervised (i.e. system operation was fully autonomous) in a washroom for a day program for people with dementia (Czarnuch *et al.*, 2013). These trials demonstrated the ability of autonomous technology to assist people with dementia while also identifying the next areas in need of development; notably, more robust computer vision algorithms for hand tracking, and a greater ability for COACH to interpret context. Work is underway on the next version of

COACH, which is intended to be installed in people's homes for long-term trials. In addition to expanding the boundaries of applied computer science, the COACH project expanded to include implementation on a personal robotics platform (Begum *et al.*, 2013) and adaption for children with autism spectrum disorder (Bimbrahw *et al.*, 2012). Other areas of research inspired by experiences with COACH trials include the investigation of how tap design impacts usability by people with dementia (Boger *et al.*, 2013), the use of actors to simulate people with dementia in order to optimize technologies prior to deployment in trials with real participants (Boger *et al.*, 2010), and the analysis of communication strategies used by caregivers when assisting with activity completion (Wilson *et al.*, 2012).

Ideally, interventions for people with dementia will help to slow or halt cognitive decline, thereby preserving as much psychomotor function as possible. Some ATCs are attempting to achieve this by enabling enjoyable activities that stimulate cognition. One example is the work done by Martin and colleagues (Martin *et al.*, 2013) that uses social robotics as a form of cognitive stimulation therapy. The researchers programmed a Nao humanoid robot with language, music therapy, storytelling, and physiotherapy sessions that were developed by therapists and clinicians with expertise in dementia. The robot was tested through a month of twice-weekly therapy sessions with 13 participants with moderate-to-severe dementia. Participants appeared to enjoy interacting with the robot and trended toward improvements in neuropsychiatric symptoms, apathy, and quality of life. Therapists manually triggered robotic actions, but it is conceivable that the robot could be automated in the future. Another example of a device to support leisure activities is ePAD, which is a touch-screen canvas that supports arts therapy with people with dementia. Created by Leuty and colleagues (Leuty *et al.*, 2012), the goal of ePAD is to enable arts therapists to develop and share customized arts programs with their clients. As a person with dementia interacts with ePAD's multi-touch surface, it is able to estimate his or her level of engagement autonomously, and play cues, such as sounds or displaying images, to the canvas to help encourage participation in the art creation process if the user is becoming disengaged. ePAD is able to save sessions so they can be reviewed by therapists, the people with dementia, and their families, as well as track metrics that give therapists objective measures of how clients interacted with the canvas. Trials with six people with dementia and their therapists concluded that ePAD was engaging and interesting for both therapists and their clients; however, the usefulness of the autonomous prompting was not clear. The researchers plan to investigate whether the autonomous prompting feature could be improved or whether there are other features that would be more useful.

Robot-guided post-stroke movement rehabilitation

Stroke affects 16.3 million people worldwide every year and is the leading cause of acquired physical disability and one of the leading causes of death (Truelsen and Bonita, 2009). Blockages or lesions to blood vessels deprive areas of the brain of oxygen and glucose, resulting in permanent damage to brain tissues. The effects of a stroke depend on what part of the brain was damaged and the severity of the damage, with motor, speech, vision, and behavior often compromised. Partial or full paralysis of a limb is common, with upper extremities typically more affected than lower extremities (Adams, 2007). While medical treatments are becoming increasingly effective for acute treatment of stroke, there is often residual damage (Donnan et al., 2008). Over time, a stroke survivor may undergo a partial or full recovery of abilities if his or her brain is able to reroute neural activity around the damaged area or repurpose other areas of the brain. Maximizing post-stroke recovery is a complex process that requires assessment and treatment by a multidisciplinary team, including physiotherapy, occupational therapy, speech therapy, nutritional assessment, psychology, and social services (Summers et al., 2009; Lang et al., 2011). Access to rehabilitation therapy has been shown to be key to recovery, resulting in a decrease in the severity of both acute and long-term impairments caused by stroke. Research suggests that the earlier and more focused the rehabilitation intervention is, the greater the potential functional gains are (Langhorne et al., 2009). Moreover, relevant task-specific and context-specific exercises that motivate the stroke survivor tend to result in better motor learning outcomes (Langhorne et al., 2011).

One form of conventional physical therapy is repetitive task training, which consists of repetitive movement of the affected limb in a targeted, controlled manner to relearn and regain precision and range of motion (Langhorne et al., 2011). While it has been shown that a stroke survivor should have unlimited access to therapy to achieve the best possible outcomes, there is often a limited number of therapists available. *Rehabilitation robotics* is looking to bridge this gap by providing a means of guided repetitive motion therapy. In addition to providing greater access to therapy, well-designed systems could provide activities that make rehabilitation exercises more fun, meaningful, and engaging. Robotic-guided therapy also has the ability to measure rehabilitation progress empirically in an objective fashion, which could provide valuable metrics to the therapists and motivation for people undergoing therapy (Reinkensmeyer and Boninger, 2012).

About 80 percent of stroke survivors will be able to walk again, while only 55 to 75 percent regain upper-limb function by three to six months (Rodgers et al., 2003). As a result, there have been many robotic interventions aimed at upper-limb rehabilitation. One of the best known and most thoroughly evaluated systems is the MIT–Manus, which has been in development over the past two decades (Krebs et al., 2003). MIT-Manus aims to rehabilitate gross motor movement by having a user move the end-effector of a robotic arm in directions indicated on a computer screen. In a study involving 127 participants, MIT-Manus assisted participants showed significantly better results compared to participants who received usual post-stroke care and no difference compared to a group that received intensive therapy (Lo et al., 2010). This suggests upper-limb robotic-guided therapy can be equivalent to intensive human-guided efforts, which is a significant finding as most stroke survivors are not able to access this level of treatment currently.

Ideally, rehabilitation robots should be in a form that is portable and affordable (i.e. can be rented from a hospital or purchased outright) so that they are available for in-home use, enabling a stroke survivor to engage rehabilitation in a familiar setting whenever and as often as he or she wishes (Andrade *et al.*, 2014). A transdisciplinary team of researchers from the University of Toronto teamed up with an industrial partner, Quanser (a company that specializes in control systems and robotics), to create a robot that can be set up on a table top (Huq *et al.*, 2013; Kan *et al.*, 2011). The robot is capable of delivering haptic feedback; namely, forces that reflect what a user is seeing on a screen (e.g. making a user feel like they are being pulled toward a target or pushed away from an obstacle), thereby adding a dimension of tactile feedback to exercises. While this is not the first portable rehabilitation robot, what is exceptional is that it uses AI to autonomously estimate factors such as user fatigue, and uses this information to alter the exercises dynamically in real-time to match changes in the user's ability. In this way, the therapist and robot work as a team, with therapists providing high-level guidance and supervision of rehabilitation progress while the robot manages changes within each session. Pilot trials have shown promising results, but the robot has yet to be evaluated in clinical trials with stroke survivors, which are scheduled to begin in autumn of 2014.

While robotic rehabilitation is an intriguing and promising addition to motion-based rehabilitation, it is still not clear what role robots will play. As put by Reinkensmeyer *et al.* (2007: 1012), "we know that effort, engagement, and error matter for motor recovery. For a rehabilitation robot, promoting engagement and effort may be as simple as providing ongoing feedback about the patient's participation". Currently, the best robot-assisted therapy does not achieve better results than conventional (human-guided) therapy, but it does perform comparably (Mehrholz *et al.*, 2012; Norouzi-Gheidari *et al.*, 2012). As robotic systems become cheaper, and AI becomes more advanced, robotic-guided therapy may one day surpass human-guided, in terms of both availability and outcomes. For comprehensive overviews and examples of upper- and lower-limb rehabilitation robotics, see the reviews by Loureiro *et al.* (2011), Díaz *et al.* (2011), Turchetti *et al.* (2014), and Maciejasz *et al.* (2014).

Conclusions

The ever-expanding capabilities of hardware and software, including the introduction of pervasive (ubiquitous) computing, mean that applications are beginning to be limited only by our imaginations. The examples presented in this chapter discusses just a few of the populations and contexts that could benefit from ITCs. While a great deal of progress has been made, there is still a tremendous amount of research that needs to be done. Most ITCs are currently stand-alone platforms; communication, data sharing, and privacy protocols are just some of the areas that need to be developed and standardized before integrated, ubiquitous systems are possible. Beyond the inherent technical hurdles, creating an ITC is a challenging endeavor as users' abilities, preferences, and environments are profoundly different from one another, yet effective support must complement each individual's circumstances. In each case, it is necessary to gain an understanding of the contexts of the intended application, including what sort of intervention should be used and how it impacts the people who are using it. Thus, creating valuable interventions necessitates close collaboration between experts in many fields, including computer science, rehabilitation science, engineering, medicine, and, of course, representative end-users.

For an intervention to be truly useful, it must consistently achieve its intended goal in a way that is acceptable and, ideally, effortless. It cannot be stressed enough that, while high-tech interventions have significant potential, there are many very effective low-tech solutions. For example, using bright, contrasting colors and familiar objects can greatly improve the day-to-day performance of older adults with dementia because this intuitively makes their environment more usable for them (e.g. van Hoof *et al.*, 2010; Boger *et al.*, 2013). Adapting and combining support techniques, artificially intelligent and otherwise, lies at the heart of enabling people with compromised psychomotor abilities to participate meaningfully in their lives. Moreover, it is vitally important that the dignity and wellbeing of the people supported by the intervention are respected, including choosing what technology to use and when to use it. This is just as important in cases where it can be difficult for the intended end user to articulate their wishes, such as a person with dementia or a child with autism spectrum disorder.

There is still much work to do before the examples discussed in this chapter are ready for the consumer market; however, they do represent ways that technology is advancing the paradigm of healthcare delivery, and give us a feel for what is to come in the not-too-distant future. It is hoped that this chapter has provided a glimpse into the remarkable realm of high-tech ATCs for supporting psychomotor functioning, including an appreciation for the exciting transdisciplinary research challenges that lie ahead.

References

Adams, H. P. J. (2007). *Principles of Cerebrovascular Disease*. New York, NY: McGraw-Hill.

Andrade, A. O., Pereira, A. A., Walter, S., Almeida, R., Loureiro, R., Compagna, D., and Kyberd, P. J. (2014). Bridging the Gap Between Robotic Technology and Health Care. *Biomedical Signal Processing and Control*, 10: 65–78.

Begum, M., Wang, R., Huq, R., and Mihailidis, A. (2013). Performance of Daily Activities by Older Adults with Dementia: The Role of an Assistive Robot. *IEEE International Conference on Rehabilitation Robotics*, June 24–6, Seattle, WA.

Bimbrahw, J., Boger, J., and Mihailidis, A. (2012). Investigating the Efficacy of a Computerized Prompting Device to Assist Children with Autism Spectrum Disorder with Activities of Daily Living. *Assistive Technology*, 24(4): 286–98.

Boger, J., Hoey, J., Poupart, P., Boutilier, C., Fernie, G., and Mihailidis, A. (2006). A Planning System based on Markov Decision Processes to Guide People with Dementia through Activities of Daily Living. *IEEE Transactions on Information Technology in Biomedicine*, 10(2): 323–33.

Boger, J., Fenton, K., Craig, T., and Mihailidis, A. (2010). Using Actors to Develop Technologies for Older Adults with Dementia: A Pilot Study. *Gerontechnology*, 9(4): 57–74.

Boger, J., Craig, T., and Mihailidis, A. (2013). Examining the Impact of Familiarity on Faucet Usability for Older Adults with Dementia. *BMC Geriatrics*, 13. Available at: www.biomedcentral.com/1471-2318/13/63 (accessed 26 September 2014).

Boucher, P., Atrash, A., Kelouwani, S., Honore, W., Nguyen, H., Villemure, J., Routhier, F., Cohen, P., Demers, L., Forget, R., and Pineau, J. (2013). Design and Validation of an Intelligent Wheelchair Towards a Clinically-Functional Outcome. *Journal of NeuroEngineering and Rehabilitation*, 10: 58.

Bourret, E. M., Bernick, L. G., Cott, C. A., and Kontos, P. C. (2002). The Meaning of Mobility for Residents and Staff in Long-Term Care Facilities. *Journal of Advanced Nursing*, 37: 338–45.

Bruvik, F. K., Ulstein, I. D., Ranhoff, A. H., and Engedal, K. (2013). The Effect of Coping on the Burden in Family Carers of Persons with Dementia. *Aging and Mental Health*, 17(8): 973–78.

Clyburn, L. D., Stones, M. J., Hadjistavropoulos, T., and Tuokko, H. (2000). Predicting Caregiver Burden and Depression in Alzheimer's Disease. *Journals of Gerontology Series B: Psychological Sciences and Social Sciences*, 55: S2–S13.

Craig, D., Mirakhur, A., Hart, D. J., Mcilroy, S. P., and Passmore, A. P. (2005). A Cross-Sectional Study of Neuropsychiatric Symptoms in 435 Patients with Alzheimer's Disease. *The American Journal of Geriatric Psychiatry*, 13: 460–8.

Czarnuch, S., Cohen, S., Parameswaran, V., and Mihailidis, A. (2013). A Real-World Deployment of the COACH Prompting System. *Journal of Ambient Intelligence and Smart Environments*, 5(5): 463–78.

Daviglus, M. L., Bell, C. C., Berrettini, W., Bowen, P. E., Connolly, J. E. S., Cox, N. J., Dunbar-Jacob, J. M., Granieri, E. C., Hunt, G., Mcgarry, K., Patel, D., Potosky, A. L., Sanders-Bush, E., Silberberg, D., and Trevisan, M. (2010). National Institutes of Health State-of-the-Science Conference Statement: Preventing Alzheimer's Disease and Cognitive Decline. *Annals of Internal Medicine*, 153: 176–81.

Díaz, I., Gil, J. J., and Sánchez, E. (2011). Lower-limb Robotic Rehabilitation: Literature Review and Challenges. *Journal of Robotics*, 2011: 1–11. Available at: www.hindawi.com/journals/jr/2011/759764/ (accessed 26 September 2014).

Dickie, V. (2009). What is Occupation? In Crepeau, E. B., Cohn, E. S., and Boyt Schell, B. A. (eds), *Willard and Spackman's Occupational Therapy*. Philadelphia, PA: Wolters Kluwer/Lippincott, Williams & Wilkins.

Donnan, G. A., Fisher, M., Macleod, M., and Davis, S. M. (2008). Stroke. *The Lancet*, 371: 1612–23.

Fetherstonhaugh, D., Tarzia, L., and Nay, R. (2013). Being Central to Decision Making Means I am Still Here! The Essence of Decision Making for People with Dementia. *Journal of Aging Studies*, 27: 143–50.

Galway, L., O'Neill, S., Donnelly, M., Nugent, C., McClean, S., and Scotney, B., (2013). Stakeholder Involvement Guidelines to Improve the Design Process of Assistive Technology: Lessons from the Development of the MPVS System. *Health and Technology*, 3(2): 119–27.

Hoey, J., Poupart, P., Bertoldi, A., Craig, T., Boutilier, C., and Mihailidis, A. (2010). Automated Handwashing Assistance for Persons with Dementia using Video and a Partially Observable Markov Decision Process. *Computer Vision and Image Understanding*, 114(5): 503–19.

How, T. -V., Wang, R. H., and Mihailidis, A. (2013). Evaluation of an Intelligent Wheelchair System for Older Adults with Cognitive Impairments. *Journal of NeuroEngineering and Rehabilitation*, 10: 90.

Huq, R., Wang, R., Lu, E., Hebert, D., Lacheray, H., and Mihailidis, A., (2013). Development of a Fuzzy Logic Based Intelligent System for Autonomous Guidance of Post-stroke Rehabilitation Exercise. *IEEE International Conference on Rehabilitation Robotics*, June 24–26 (pp. 1–8), Seattle, WA.

Kan, P., Huq, R., Hoey, J., Goetschalckx, R., and Mihailidis, A. (2011). The Development of an Adaptive Upper-Limb Stroke Rehabilitation Robotic System. *Journal of Neuro-Engineering and Rehabilitation*, 8(1): 1–18.

Kirby, R. L., Dupuis, D. J., Macphee, A. H., Coolen, A. L., Smith, C., Best, K. L., Newton, A. M., Mountain, A. D., Macleod, D. A., and Bonaparte, J. P. (2004). The Wheelchair Skills Test (Version 2.4): Measurement Properties. *Archives of Physical Medicine and Rehabilitation*, 85: 794–804.

Kluger, A., Gianutsos, J. G., Golomb, J., Ferris, S. H., George, A. E., Franssen, E., and Reisberg, B. (1997). Patterns of Motor Impairment in Normal Aging, Mild Cognitive Decline, and Early Alzheimer's Disease. *The Journals of Gerontology Series B: Psychological Sciences and Social Sciences*, 52B: P28–P39.

Krebs, H. I., Palazzolo, J. J., Dipietro, L., Ferraro, M., Krol, J., Rannekleiv, K., Volpe, B. T., and Hogan, N. (2003). Rehabilitation Robotics: Performance-Based Progressive Robot-Assisted Therapy. *Autonomous Robots*, 15: 7–20.

Lang, C. E., Bland, M. D., Connor, L. T., Fucetola, R., Whitson, M., Edmiaston, J., Karr, C., Sturmoski, A., Baty, J., and Corbetta, M. (2011). The Brain Recovery Core: Building a System of Organized Stroke Rehabilitation and Outcomes Assessment Across the Continuum of Care. *Journal of Neurologic Physical Therapy*, 35: 194–201.

Langhorne, P., Coupar, F., and Pollock, A. (2009). Motor Recovery after Stroke: A Systematic Review. *The Lancet Neurology*, 8: 741–54.

Langhorne, P., Bernhardt, J., and Kwakkel, G. (2011). Stroke Rehabilitation. *The Lancet*, 377: 1693–702.

Leuty, V., Boger, J. N., Young, L., Hoey, J., and Mihailidis, A. (2012). Engaging Older Adults with Dementia in Creative Occupations Using Artificially Intelligent Assistive Technology. *Assistive Technology*, 25(2): 72–9.

Lo, A. C., Guarino, P. D., Richards, L. G., Haselkorn, J. K., Wittenberg, G. F., Federman, D. G., Ringer, R. J., Wagner, T. H., Krebs, H. I., Volpe, B. T., Bever, C. T., Bravata, D. M., Duncan, P. W., Corn, B. H., Maffucci, A. D., Nadeau, S. E., Conroy, S. S., Powell, J. M., Huang, G. D., and Peduzzi, P. (2010). Robot-Assisted Therapy for Long-Term Upper-Limb Impairment after Stroke. *New England Journal of Medicine*, 362: 1772–83.

Loureiro, R. C., Harwin, W. S., Nagai, K., and Johnson, M. (2011). Advances in Upper Limb Stroke Rehabilitation: A Technology Push. *Medical and Biological Engineering and Computing*, 49(10): 1103–18.

Maciejasz, P., Eschweiler, J., Gerlach-Hahn, K., Jansen-Troy, A., and Leonhardt, S. (2014). A Survey on Robotic Devices for Upper Limb Rehabilitation. *Journal of NeuroEngineering and Rehabilitation*, 11(1): 3.

Martin, F., Aguero, C., Canas, J. M., Abella, G., Benitez, R., Rivero, S., Valenti, M., and Martinez-Martin, P. (2013). Robots in Therapy for Dementia Patients. *Journal of Physical Agents*, 7(1): 48–55.

Mehrholz, J., Hädrich, A., Platz, T., Kugler, J., and Pohl, M. (2012). Electromechanical and Robot-Assisted Arm Training for Improving Generic Activities of Daily Living, Arm Function and Arm Muscle Strength after Stroke. *Cochrane Database of Systematic Reviews*, 13(6): CD006876.

Merriam-Webster (2014). Merriam-Webster medical dictionary. http://www.merriam-webster.com/ (accessed 26 September 2014).

Metz, D. H. (2000). Mobility of Older People and their Quality of Life. *Transport Policy*, 7: 149–52.

Mihailidis, A., Fernie, G. R., and Barbenel, J. C. (2001). The Use of Artificial Intelligence in the Design of an Intelligent Cognitive Orthosis for People with Dementia. *Assistive Technology*, 13(1): 23–39.

Mihailidis, A., Boger, J., Canido, M., and Hoey, J. (2008a). The Use of an Intelligent Prompting System for People with Dementia. *Interactions*, 14(4): 34–7.

Mihailidis, A., Boger, J. N., Craig, T., and Hoey, J. (2008b). The COACH Prompting System to Assist Older Adults with Dementia through Handwashing: An Efficacy Study. *BMC Geriatrics*, 8(1): 28.

Mihailidis, A., Boger, J., Hoey, J., and Jiancaro, T. (2011). Zero Effort Technologies: Considerations, Challenges and Use in Health, Wellness and Rehabilitation. In Baecker, R. M. (ed.), *Synthesis Lectures on Assistive, Rehabilitative, and Health-Preserving Technologies*. San Rafael, CA: Morgan & Claypool Publishers.

Mortenson, W. B., Miller, W. C., Boily, J., Steele, B., Crawford, E. M., and Desharnais, G. (2006). Overarching Principles and Salient Findings for Inclusion in Guidelines for Power Mobility Use within Residential Care Facilities. *Journal of Rehabilitation Research and Development*, 43: 199–208.

Norouzi-Gheidari, N., Archambault, P. S., and Fung, J. (2012). Effects of Robot-Assisted Therapy on Stroke Rehabilitation in Upper Limbs: Systematic Review and Meta-analysis of the Literature. *Journal of Rehabilitation Research and Development*, 49(4): 479–96.

O'Neill, S. A., Parente, G., Donnelly, M. P., Nugent, C. D., Boyd, K. A., McClean, S., Scotney, B., Mason, S., and Craig, D., (2011). Incorporation of Carer and Patient Needs in the Development of Assistive Technology for People with Dementia. In Anderson, M. (ed.), *Contemporary Ergonomics and Human Factors 2011; Proceedings of the International Conference on Ergonomics and Human Factors 2011*, Stoke Rochford Hall, Lincolnshire, April 12–14. CRC Press.

O'Neill, S., McClean, S., Donnelly, M., Nugent, C., Galway, L., Cleland, I., Zhang, S., Young, T., Scotney, B., Mason, S., and Craig, D. (2014). Development of a Technology Adoption and Usage Prediction Tool for Assistive Technology for People with Dementia. *Interacting with Computers*, 26(2): 169–76.

Peula, J. M., Urdiales, C., Herrero, I., Fernandez-Carmona, M., and Sandoval, F. (2012). Case-Based Reasoning Emulation of Persons for Wheelchair Navigation. *Artificial Intelligence in Medicine*, 56: 109–21.

Proctor, R. W. and Dutta, A. (1995). *Skill Acquisition and Human Performance*. Thousand Oaks, CA: Sage.

Reinkensmeyer, D. and Boninger, M. (2012). Technologies and Combination Therapies for Enhancing Movement Training for People with a Disability. *Journal of NeuroEngineering and Rehabilitation*, 9: 17.

Reinkensmeyer, D. J., Galvez, J. A., Marchal, L., Wolbrecht, E. T., and Bobrow, J. E. (2007). Some Key Problems for Robot-Assisted Movement Therapy Research: A Perspective from the University of California at Irvine. In *IEEE 10th International Conference on Rehabilitation Robotics*, June 13–15 (pp. 1009–15).

Rodgers, H., Mackintosh, J., Price, C., Wood, R., Mcnamee, P., Fearon, T., Marritt, A., and Curless, R. (2003). Does an Early Increased-Intensity Interdisciplinary Upper Limb Therapy Programme Following Acute Stroke Improve Outcome? *Clinical Rehabilitation*, 17: 579–89.

Russell, S. J. and Norvig, P. (2010). *Artificial Intelligence: A Modern Approach* (third edition). Upper Saddle River, NJ: Prentice Hall.

Sathian, K., Buxbaum, L. J., Cohen, L. G., Krakauer, J. W., Lang, C. E., Corbetta, M., and Fitzpatrick, S. M. (2011). Neurological Principles and Rehabilitation of Action Disorders: Common Clinical Deficits. *NeuroRehabilitation and Neural Repair*, 25(5): 21S–32S.

Scherer, M. J., Sax, C., Vanbeirvliet, A., Cushman, L. A., and Scherer, J. V. (2005). Predictors of Assistive Technology Use: The Importance of Personal and Psychosocial Factors. *Disability and Rehabilitation*, 27(21): 1321–31.

Schulz, R., Beach, S. R., Matthews, J. T., Courtney, K., Devito Dabbs, A., Person Mecca, L., and Scott Sankey, S. (2012). Willingness to Pay for Quality of Life Technologies to Enhance Independent Functioning among Baby Boomers and the Elderly Adults. *The Gerontologist*, 54(3): 363–74.

Shah, S. G., Robinson, I., and AlShawi, S. (2009). Developing Medical Device Technologies from Users' Perspectives: A Theoretical Framework for Involving Users in the Development Process. *International Journal of Technology Assessment in Health Care*, 25(4): 514–21.

Simpson, R. C. (2005). Smart Wheelchairs: A Literature Review. *Journal of Rehabilitation Research and Development*, 42: 423–38.

Simpson, R. C., LoPresti, E. F., and Cooper, R. A. (2008). How Many People Would Benefit from a Smart Wheelchair? *Journal of Rehabilitation Research and Development*, 45: 53–72.

Spinney, J. E. L., Scott, D. M., and Newbold, K. B. (2009). Transport Mobility Benefits and Quality of Life: A Time-Use Perspective of Elderly Canadians. *Transport Policy*, 16: 1–11.

Summers, D., Leonard, A., Wentworth, D., Saver, J. L., Simpson, J., Spilker, J. A., Hock, N., Miller, E., and Mitchell, P. H. (2009). Comprehensive Overview of Nursing and Interdisciplinary Care of the Acute Ischemic Stroke Patient. *Stroke*, 40: 2911–44.

Torti, F. M. J., Gwyther, L. P., Reed, S. D., Friedman, J. Y., and Schulman, K. A. (2004). A Multinational Review of Recent Trends and Reports in Dementia Caregiver Burden. *Alzheimer Disease and Associated Disorders*, 18: 99–109.

Townsend, E. (1997). Occupation: Potential for Personal and Social Transformation. *Journal of Occupational Science*, 4: 18–26.

Truelsen, T. and Bonita, R. (2009). Handbook of Clinical Neurology. In Fisher, M. (ed.), *Stroke Part I: Basic and Epidemiological Aspects*. Amsterdam, the Netherlands: Elsevier.

Turchetti, G., Vitiello, N., Trieste, L., Romiti, S., Geisler, E., and Micera, S. (2014). Why Effectiveness of Robot-Mediated Neuro-Rehabilitation does not Necessarily Influence its Adoption. *IEEE Reviews in Biomedical Engineering*, 7: 143–53.

Urdiales, C., Fernández-Carmona, M., Peula, J. M., Cortés, U., Annichiaricco, R., Caltagirone, C., and Sandoval, F. (2011). Wheelchair Collaborative Control for Disabled Users Navigating Indoors. *Artificial Intelligence in Medicine*, 52: 177–91.

Üstün, T. B., Chatterji, S., Bickenbach, J., Kostanjsek, N., and Schneider, M. (2003). The International Classification of Functioning, Disability and Health: A New Tool for Understanding Disability and Health. *Disability and Rehabilitation*, 25: 565–71.

Van Hoof, J., Kort, H. S. M., Van Waarde, H., and Blom, M. M. (2010). Environmental Interventions and the Design of Homes for Older Adults with Dementia: An Overview. *American Journal of Alzheimer's Disease and Other Dementias*, 25: 202–32.

Viswanathan, P., Little, J., Mackworth, A., and Mihailidis, A. (2011). Navigation and Obstacle Avoidance Help (NOAH) for Older Adults with Cognitive Impairment: A Pilot Study. In *ACM SIGACCESS Conference on Computers and Accessibility (ASSETS)*, 2011, Dundee, Scotland.

Viswanathan, P., Little, J. J., Mackworth, A. K., and Mihailidis, A. (2012). An Intelligent Powered Wheelchair for Users with Dementia: Case Studies with NOAH (Navigation and Obstacle Avoidance Help). *AAAI Technical Report FS-12-01, Artificial Intelligence for Gerontechnology*. Available at: www.aaai.org/ocs/index.php/FSS/FSS12 (accessed 26 September 2014).

Wilson, R., Rochon, E., Mihailidis, A., and Leonard, C. (2012). Examining Success of Communication Strategies used by Formal Caregivers Assisting Individuals with

Alzheimer's Disease during an Activity of Daily Living. *Journal of Speech, Language and Hearing Research*, 55(2): 328–41.

World Health Organization (2002). *Towards a Common Language for Functioning, Disability and Health* (ICF). Geneva. Available at: www.who.int/classifications/icf/site/beginners/bg.pdf (accessed 26 September 2014).

World Health Organization (2012). *Dementia: A Public Health Priority*. Available at: http://apps.who.int/iris/bitstream/10665/75263/1/9789241564458_eng.pdf?ua=1 (accessed 26 September 2014).

10

COGNITIVE TECHNOLOGIES FOR WAYFINDING

Mark Harniss, Pat A. Brown, and Kurt L. Johnson

Although almost everyone has been temporarily lost at some point, a significant number of people have persistent difficulty in navigating a route and, when they are lost, are unable to find their way without assistance. Many of these individuals have cognitive disabilities, which affect not just their wayfinding ability, but also other important life skills as well (e.g. planning, scheduling). The American Community Survey estimates that 3.9 percent of the civilian non-institutionalized population (over 2 million people) has cognitive difficulties (US Census Bureau, 2014). Unfortunately, prevalence estimates do not exist that would tell us how many of these people experience difficulty with wayfinding. We do know that challenges in wayfinding can negatively affect an individual's ability to work, recreate, and participate in community life. For example, when an individual is unable to wayfind independently, it reduces opportunities for engagement with friends (e.g. it makes it difficult to meet your friends out at the cinema to watch a movie on the spur of the moment), for gainful employment (e.g. it makes it difficult to show up at your place of work on time), and to engage in leisure activities (e.g. it is difficult to run up the street to the soccer field for a quick game).

As we have worked to develop technologies to support wayfinding, we have found that many individuals who have difficulty with wayfinding report that they feel isolated and unable to leave home because they, or their parents and caregivers, fear the consequences of being lost. As a result, challenges in wayfinding result in a significant loss in independence and social contact because people with cognitive disabilities require support (usually from other people – parents, siblings, caregivers, para-transit) in order to travel accurately and safely.

Although supports for getting from one place to another may exist in a community, they come with significant costs in terms of flexibility and expediency. Relying on a caregiver or parent to provide transportation means that an individual is restricted to the days and times that that individual is available. Relying on a community service, such as adapted public transportation, increases one's ability to travel independently, but still comes with costs in time and flexibility since one must schedule the service in advance and often wait during a 1–2 hour window of time for the transport to arrive. Because of these challenges, many research groups have explored ways to provide technological support to people with cognitive disabilities so they may travel independently, but safely, without the need for ongoing human support.

As a component of a support system for individuals with cognitive disabilities, cognitive support technologies for wayfinding have great potential to increase independence and reduce the need for personal assistance. Like other assistive technology systems, they consist of "someone (person with a disability) doing something (an activity) somewhere (within a context)" (Cook and Polgar, 2007: 35). Thus, cognitive support technologies comprise a complex interaction between the human user, the activities in which she or he wants to engage, the context in which the activity occurs, and the assistive technology available to support the activity. Planning for the development, selection, implementation, continued use, and evaluation of cognitive support technologies requires an understanding of each variable (Scherer and Craddock, 2002).

In this chapter, we discuss the activity of wayfinding and the issues it poses for people with cognitive disabilities and then overview the technological innovations that are in development to support their independence in wayfinding. We conclude with suggestions for both clinicians and developers.

What is wayfinding?

Wayfinding refers to the ability to find one's way from a base location to another location (or locations) of interest and back again. Wayfinding can be simple (a child finding his way home from the elementary school down the block) or complex (a taxi cab driver finding her way through the streets of London to a new address). Most people use their wayfinding skills on a daily basis – to navigate to familiar places (e.g. work, school, shopping) and to novel locations (e.g. a new doctor's appointment).

Wayfinding is a foundational life skill that most humans begin to develop at a very early age. Research suggests that wayfinding develops gradually over time from an egocentric (person-based stimulus-response) approach to an allocentric (world-based place learning) approach. Children as young as nine months begin to show some use of allocentric strategies, which may be related to the development of mobility through crawling (Bremmer, 1978). Interestingly, Wiedenbauer and Jansen-Osmann (2006) have demonstrated that the age at which a child with spina bifida learns to walk strongly correlates with how many learning trials it took to acquire a route, suggesting again that mobility may be a covariate in the development of wayfinding capabilities. Development of allocentric representations appears to continue until about the age of 10 (Lehnung *et al.*, 1998; Overman *et al.*, 1996; Piajet and Inhelder, 1948). The work of Bohbot *et al.* (2012) suggests that, over the course of the lifespan, older adults (e.g. mid-60s) may revert to a more response-based wayfinding style as they automatize frequently repeated behavior.

Conceptually, wayfinding is complex, and a complete taxonomy of all the cognitive underpinnings that support successful wayfinding has yet to be developed. Researchers have classified wayfinding in different ways, including by the types of navigational knowledge that a person could possess (i.e. landmark, route, survey) and the types of wayfinding tasks in which they might engage (e.g. familiar versus unfamiliar). In the following sections, we briefly describe these classifications.

Types of knowledge

Siegel and White (1975) postulated a framework that included three types of knowledge used for navigation: landmark, route, and survey. In landmark-based navigation, individuals use recognizable features of the environment as a directional cue. Landmarks can cue an individual to move toward or away from the landmark or to implement an action (e.g. turn right) when arriving at the landmark. Landmark-based navigation does not require an overall understanding of the route, just the ability to identify a landmark and execute an action when the landmark is reached. Obviously, not all landmarks are equal (Chan *et al.*, 2012). We have found that the difficulty of using a landmark in navigation can vary depending upon the type of landmark (e.g. building, school, sculpture, road), the uniqueness of the landmark, the distance between the individual and the landmark, the orientation of the landmark to the individual (e.g. in front, behind, to the left or right), and the alignment of the landmark to the path (e.g. walk toward versus keep to your left) (Liu *et al.*, 2009).

Route knowledge refers to navigation that relies on place–action associations. These place–actions can include landmarks, but may also include other types of information (e.g. distance and cardinal direction – for example, "walk down 4th Street for 4 blocks until you reach the clock tower, then turn left"). Neither landmark nor route knowledge requires an individual to have a cognitive map of the environment.

Survey-level knowledge refers to the type of navigation in which an individual has a higher level understanding of the environment that may include a cognitive map of the area with a sense for how routes fit together and the specific distances and angles between locations. Landmark and route knowledge are considered to be egocentric frames of reference because they require navigation that is from the person-level or ground-level perspective. Survey-level knowledge is considered to be an allocentric frame of reference because it requires the individual to hold a frame of reference or perspective that is independent of his or her current location (Klatzky, 1998).

Recently, Chrastil (2013) discussed the adequacy of this three-part framework. She noted that, although the framework makes conceptual sense, it is not empirically-based, does not map to distinct neural correlates, and each type of knowledge likely involves multiple cognitive processes. She argues that, "a finer-grained breakdown of the cognitive processes and sub-processes involved in spatial knowledge is in order" (2013: 210). As part of this effort, she proposed a fourth type of navigational knowledge that she called graph knowledge. Graph knowledge fits between route and survey levels of knowledge and refers to navigation through an understanding of connected points in space (i.e. topological connections) that could be represented like a network map. This type of knowledge is more sophisticated than route knowledge, in which a navigator only knows one path to a destination, but less sophisticated than survey-level knowledge, in which a navigator has an accurate (metric) representation of all possible routes.

Types of wayfinding tasks

In addition to types of knowledge required, wayfinding tasks can also be categorized by type of task. Wayfinding tasks may be made easier or harder depending upon whether the wayfinding is aided or unaided, whether the route is familiar or unfamiliar, and whether the trip is planned or unplanned (Wiener et al., 2009). Aid can come in many forms, both human and technological, but is often required by individuals with cognitive disabilities, especially if they are going somewhere unfamiliar or the trip is unplanned. When routes are unfamiliar or unplanned, most people engage in exploratory activities (e.g. wandering around a new school campus or exploring a new neighborhood) that allow them to develop an understanding of the environment in which they are traveling; however, for people with cognitive disabilities exploration can be risky and non-productive. In our work, we have found that many people with cognitive disability find themselves limited to traveling to familiar places for planned trips, often with the assistance of a human caregiver.

How does cognitive disability affect wayfinding?

People with cognitive impairments are not a homogeneous group and the disabilities they experience have diverse etiologies. Wayfinding research has been conducted with people with cognitive disabilities as a result of atypical development (i.e. intellectual/developmental disabilities such as Down's syndrome, Williams' syndrome, autistic spectrum disorders, and spina bifida) (Courbois et al., 2013a; Courbois et al., 2013b; Farran et al., 2012; Lind et al., 2013; Mengue-Topio et al., 2011; Wiedenbauer and Jansen-Osmann, 2006), injury (e.g. traumatic brain injury, cerebrovascular accident/stroke) (Lemoncello et al., 2010; van der Ham et al., 2013), degenerative conditions (e.g. multiple sclerosis) (Fong et al., 2006; Uc et al., 2007), and aging (both typical aging and conditions associated with aging such as dementia) (Deipolyi et al., 2007; Head and Isom, 2010; Iaria et al., 2009).

Across disability categories, the evidence tends to suggest that people with cognitive disabilities rely on landmark knowledge over other types of knowledge, but may not identify or remember the best landmarks. With good instruction, they learn to execute routes with fluency, but make more errors during initial learning, take more time, and are more hesitant in execution of the route. Finally, although they may develop survey-level knowledge, their cognitive maps are often less complete and more distorted. Different causes of cognitive disability are linked to different profiles or patterns of functional deficits as a result of the ways those conditions affect the neurological status of the brain. Background knowledge and experience also appear to play a role in wayfinding (Frankenstein *et al.*, 2012; Wiedenbauer and Jansen-Osmann, 2006; Woollett and Maguire, 2010): people with more opportunity to explore and learn about the logic of environments (e.g. common placement of landmarks) perform better.

It is important to note that many people with cognitive disability also have co-morbid disabilities that affect hearing, vision or mobility. This cognitive, sensory, and physical diversity has implications for the development of appropriate technologies for supporting wayfinding that we discuss in more detail in later sections of this chapter.

Cognitive support technologies for wayfinding

Providing an appropriate support system can make a substantial difference in the lives of people with disabilities. Support systems consist of three components: personal assistance services, assistive technology, and adaptive strategies (Litvak and Enders, 2001). All three are necessary and important, and no single component can provide an individual with adequate support alone. In any given situation or environment, an individual may rely more heavily on one type of support than another. Cook and Polgar (2007) describe the shifting use of support systems as functional allocation, and Litvak and Enders describe dynamic support systems, but different approaches (personal assistance, assistive technology, adaptive strategies) are optimal for different people and different tasks.

Cognitive support technologies are devices and services intended to reduce the impact of disability for individuals with functional deficits in cognition. These technologies are often referred to as assistive technology for cognition (ATC). When cognitive support technologies are implemented well, they can benefit individuals with cognitive disabilities by increasing independence and success in life activities. These technologies can also enhance the quality of life of caregivers by reducing the demands of that role.

The evidence base for cognitive support technologies for navigation and wayfinding is currently sparse. In two systematic evidence reviews published since 2010 (de Joode *et al.*, 2010; Gillespie *et al.*, 2011) only seven published studies of technologies met the minimum inclusion criteria for quality and were included in the reviews. Of these, four included participants with cognitive impairments (TBI, ABI, intellectual disabilities, MS) and three included elderly participants and those with dementia.

Gillespie *et al.* (2011) rate the evidence from the four studies of participants with cognitive impairments from 2 (well-conducted case control or cohort with a low risk of bias) to 3 (case control or cohort with a high risk of bias) using the Scottish Intercollegiate Guidelines Network (2008) methodology. De Joode *et al.* (2010) rate the evidence of two of the studies also included in the Gillespie *et al.* review as Class III, using methods described by Cicerone *et al.* (2000). Class III studies were clinical series without concurrent controls (Sohlberg *et al.*, 2007), or studies with results from one or more single cases that used appropriate single-subject methods, such as multiple baselines across interventions with adequate quantification and analysis of results (Kirsch *et al.*, 2004).

In all, the preliminary evidence indicates that user confidence and accuracy in wayfinding improves with the use of customizable cognitive support technologies for navigation. Although most devices are prototypes and not available for the general public, the work in this area has grown from using bulky, external GPS units and hand-held PDAs to customized smartphones and specialized apps.

Existing technologies

Most of the work done in the area of navigation and wayfinding has been in facilitating outdoor navigation. Outdoor navigation is based on GPS and/or cell tower positions. Technologies utilizing these systems, such as car navigation systems and apps for most smartphones, work quite well but are not error free. These systems require regular updating and, at best, location is accurate within 50 feet (Stephenson and Limbrick, 2013).

Representation in existing technologies typically includes text (step-by-step) directions with speech output and a map with directional overlay (e.g. a moving car, an arrow, or a compass) and speech output. Prompting is provided as corrective feedback when the traveler makes an error.

Existing technologies developed specifically for individuals with cognitive impairments are still largely in the pilot stages and none have been widely deployed. These cognitive support technologies specific to navigation rely on sensors in the environment for indoor navigation and GPS/cell tower positioning with human backup for outdoor navigation.

The form factors have evolved in cognitive support technologies as they have with technologies not specifically developed for individuals with disabilities. Hand-held PDAs and pagers (such as NeuroPage) have given way to apps developed for use on mobile phones for outdoor navigation. Using sensors to interpret environmental cues to location indoors, such as differences in fluorescent lighting, has evolved into using sensors embedded in the environment to locate and orient the user, such as AmbienNet (Abascal *et al.*, 2010) and AssistMote (Chang and Wang, 2010b).

Despite advances in both outdoor and indoor navigation technology, issues remain that result in barriers to use of both existing and designated devices for individuals with cognitive impairments, including reliability of location information, provision of information about orientation (i.e. "in which direction am I facing?"), representation, and prompting or cuing. In addition to these technical and user interface challenges, we have also identified barriers related to decisions about privacy, independence, and safety that arise when new technologies are put in place.

Issues in location and orientation

In outdoor navigation systems, we rely on GPS and/or cell tower positions (GSM). As noted above, these are only accurate to within approximately 50 feet. For individuals with impaired executive function resulting in difficulty with problem solving, approximate location is not adequate. Human-backed technology (Bigham et al., 2011) ensures just-in-time reliable assistance when needed. In focus groups with individuals with cognitive impairments and their caregivers (Chu et al., 2013), human-backed technology was highly valued. Participants stated that they thought technology, especially for navigation, could fail and "a real life person backup is always going to be important."

Indoor navigation also poses significant issues in location and orientation. We can determine a person's location indoors by dead reckoning (using sensors such as accelerometers to estimate current location), direct sensing (e.g. use of RFID, bar codes) or triangulation (wireless base stations in the environment) (Fallah et al., 2013). Of these, direct sensing provides the most accurate information, but requires changes in the environment (installation of the sensors) and a way for the individual to receive the information. In early pilot studies of indoor navigation (Fong et al., 2006; Liu et al., 2008; Uc et al., 2007) they determined that the use of multiple sensors for localization was essential. Wi fi, while useful, does not provide orientation and typically does not work in elevators. Combining other sensors (such as an accelerometer for dead reckoning) proves more successful in providing indoor way-finding assistance to individuals with cognitive impairments.

While technologies, especially smartphones, now have embedded sensors, such as accelerometers, recent research indicates a continued need for reliable, easily deployable, accurate indoor location and orientation technologies (Fallah et al., 2013).

Issues in representation

How information is represented, both in indoor and outdoor navigation systems, is critically important. The most common method of representation is the map. However, map usage has steadily declined in recent years; even geography students report relying on satellite navigation systems over maps to find their way in unfamiliar places (Speake and Axon, 2012). For those with some types of cognitive impairments, maps are too abstract to provide meaningful navigation assistance (Brown et al., 2005).

To address this issue, both off-the-shelf and navigation technologies developed for individuals with cognitive disabilities have trialed alternative methods of representation, including photographed landmarks and photographed landmarks with directional overlays, such as arrows (Chang and Wang, 2010a; Fong *et al.*, 2006). While landmarks selected by the end user were the most effective (Liu, 2010), individuals with intellectual disabilities have some difficulty selecting distinctive, permanent landmarks (Courbois *et al.*, 2013a). The usability of landmarks is influenced by seasonal changes (Kettunen *et al.*, 2013; Liu, 2010) prompting the recommendation in several of these studies to include either audio or text directional cues to supplement landmarks.

Issues in directional prompting

Much of our work in both indoor and outdoor navigation systems for individuals with cognitive impairments focused on effective representation and directional prompting. Lancioni *et al.* (2009) categorize directional prompting into technologies that provide corrective feedback and technologies that provide directional cues. Corrective feedback works best for individuals who are able to initiate a path, but make a mistake and need to be redirected. An early system called Opportunity Knocks (Liao *et al.*, 2007) provided corrective feedback by alerting the user to the mistake (e.g. missing a bus stop) and then providing the user with new directions to their destination.

Later iterations of Opportunity Knocks trialed the use of directional cues based on predicting where the individual is trying to go and providing guidance to the user (Liu, 2010). While we found that proactive directional cues are effective for individuals who may be unable to initiate a path, the functional variability among individuals with cognitive impairments demands a wayfinding system that is both customizable and adaptable to the end user (Liu *et al.*, 2010).

Balancing safety, privacy, and independence

As part of our research, we talked with many individuals with cognitive disabilities and their caregivers (paid and unpaid). Discussing wayfinding technologies often led them to consider the tension between the themes of safety, privacy, and independence. In short, caregivers wanted the most wayfinding independence possible for the people they supported, but worried that independence might increase risk. For example, they worried that, if their son/daughter/client were to get lost, they might end up in a neighborhood where they were at risk of predation or they might injure themselves (e.g. tip over in their wheelchair) and not be able to get assistance. However, they imagined that the technology could provide a link to allow greater independence while still maintaining the ability to monitor and provide assistance if needed.

One element of having this kind of monitoring for safety that most caregivers had not thought about much was the risk to privacy that it brought. They tended to be comfortable (especially parents) with a reduction in privacy for their son/daughter if the privacy loss was kept within the family, but had much greater concerns if the privacy loss was with an outside provider.

Discussion

Using cognitive support technologies for wayfinding in clinical practice

Implementing cognitive support technologies for wayfinding in clinical practice requires that at least two things be in place. First, there must be technologies available that are appropriate, affordable, and reliable. Second, clinicians must themselves be prepared to use, problem solve, and repair technologies as well as train consumers in the use of technologies. Unfortunately, in the field of cognitive support technologies for wayfinding, there is still much work to do before technologies can be implemented in the daily lives of people with disabilities.

Our experience suggests that commercially available devices for supporting wayfinding (GPS, smartphones, apps) are not appropriate for many people with cognitive disabilities because they are complex to operate and provide directions in ways that do not support the strengths of people with cognitive disabilities (e.g. most devices are map-oriented). There have been some improvements in recent years. For example, Garmin has developed a system called Real Directions that uses landmarks to provide directional cues. These systems may eventually be developed to a level that allows for them to be customized to the needs of people with cognitive disabilities. Individuals with cognitive disabilities who are highly motivated and have adequate support may be good candidates for trialing current systems.

Work is being done in research labs and universities to develop new technologies that are not yet commercially available. These devices, however, are not readily available to clinicians, have often only been developed to the point of proof of concept and are not reliable enough to trust with a consumer. We expect that some of the innovations being developed will eventually be built into commercially available systems, whether those systems are targeted toward the general consumer (like Garmin) or are more focused on specific populations (such as the work of companies like AbleLink).

Unfortunately, even if devices were available for use, many clinicians would not be ready to use them. De Joode et al. (2012) conducted a survey of professionals who had participated in a symposium on stroke-related cognitive rehabilitation that asked about their experience with assistive technology and opinions about its use in cognitive rehabilitation. Only about 30 percent of professionals reported previous assistive technology use. This finding suggests that not much has changed since the study conducted by Hart et al. (2003) where they found that, although clinicians believed that electronic devices could be useful in supporting their clients, especially in the areas of learning, memory, planning, and organization, two-thirds of the clinicians rated themselves as "not at all" or "somewhat" confident in their ability to teach clients how to use the devices.

Developing cognitive technologies for wayfinding for people with cognitive disabilities

Developers who want to create technologies for wayfinding that are appropriate for people with cognitive disabilities need to consider the needs and challenges of this target group. In our work, we have had the opportunity to engage in a number of user interface studies and user interviews to determine technology strategies that may work (Liu *et al.*, 2009; Liu *et al.*, 2006; Liu *et al.*, 2008). A primary recommendation we would make to developers is that they not work in isolation. They must work with consumers in a human-centered, iterative design and development process in order to understand the needs of people with cognitive disabilities and to develop effective devices.

Out of our work, we have conceptualized four design implications that developers should consider when addressing the cognitive support technology needs of people with cognitive disabilities. These four implications may help guide developers' decisions about the functionality needed in cognitive support technologies for wayfinding.

First, as a result of the differing etiologies of cognitive disabilities and varying functional limitations, we assume individuals will possess *different prerequisite skills and knowledge* that might impact the use of cognitive support technologies. For example, individuals with adult onset degenerative conditions or acquired brain injury may have been proficient technology users prior to the onset of their condition and may be able to learn to use new technology with more ease than individuals with intellectual disabilities who might not have previous experience. The design implication of these different prerequisite skill profiles is that, ideally, devices would be able to provide adaptive support for users who may need more or less assistance in learning and using the device. In addition, user interfaces will need to be developed that are intuitive and appropriate for users with diverse cognitive challenges.

Second, we expect that individuals will differ *in terms of the type of deficits with which they present*. For example, individuals with acquired brain injury may have patterns of specific and global deficits based on their specific type of injury and very specific cognitive losses related to the location of trauma, whereas individuals with intellectual disability will commonly have more generalized deficits. It is also important to remember that many individuals will present with concurrent (non-cognitive) disabilities, such as mobility or sensory impairments. The design implication of these different deficits is that devices will, ideally, be customizable (i.e. capable of being set up differently for users with different deficits – e.g. audio only for people with vision impairment, capable of supporting different input approaches for people with limited dexterity in their hands).

Third, we expect that there will be *differences in the flexibility required of the cognitive support technologies* based on an individual's condition. For example, individuals with multiple sclerosis and Alzheimer's Disease will generally have decline of cognitive function, while individuals with acquired brain injury may show improvement, and individuals with intellectual disability will likely be relatively stable in their cognitive function over time. The design implications of these different cognitive trajectories is that, ideally, a device will be adaptable over time (i.e. provide more or less support based on the user needs).

Finally, we expect that *the need for cognitive support will differ based upon the cognitive demand of the task being attempted* and that individuals who function quite well under some conditions will function less well when the demands of the task or environment change. Cognitive load theory (Paas *et al.*, 2003) acknowledges that the "cognitive architecture" of the brain (e.g. working and long-term memory, attention) has limits that can be overloaded. For example, working memory can handle only a small number of interactions at one time. When cognitive limits are reached, an individual becomes overloaded and unable to process more information. Cognitive load theorists also postulate that there are intrinsic and extraneous cognitive loads. Intrinsic loads refer to the inherent demands of the task. For example, traveling to the neighborhood store is easier than traveling to the large mall in another town. Extraneous loads are cognitive loads that serve to increase the difficulty of the task; for example, completing a trip with a time constraint or traveling during rush hour. Intrinsic load serves as the base load of the task. Extraneous load, on the other hand, is modifiable. There are many variables that can be manipulated to modify extraneous load, including novelty of the task, complexity, speed of completion, and stress. These concepts apply to individuals with disabilities using cognitive support technologies. The interrelationship between their cognitive strengths and deficits and the intrinsic and extraneous load of the task help define what an individual can do. The design implication is that cognitive technologies must provide a means for reducing, and not increasing, some of the extraneous load.

Conclusion

People with cognitive disabilities desire autonomy and self-direction as they move through the world, and they have goals and desires related to travel. However, they face challenges to autonomy that can be addressed through a good support system. Technology can serve as one element of a strong support system for wayfinding. However, there is much work to be done before these technologies are ready for "prime time." In particular, researchers need to continue research into the cognitive challenges faced by the diverse population of people with cognitive disabilities; developers need to continue working with and for people with cognitive disabilities to understand and meet their needs with creative low- and high-tech devices; and clinicians need to keep abreast of these developing technologies so they will have the skill to use them with their clients.

Acknowledgements

Work described in this chapter was funded by the US National Institute on Disability and Rehabilitation Research (NIDRR) Grant #H133A031739.

References

Abascal, J., Lafuente, A., Marco, A., Falco, J. M., Casas, R., Sevillano, J. L., and Lujan, C. (2010). An Architecture for Assisted Navigation in Intelligent Environments. *International Journal of Communication Networks and Distributed Systems*, 4(1): 49–69.

Bigham, J., Brady, E., and White, S. (2011). Human-Backed Access Technology. Paper presented at the *CHI 2011 Workshop on Crowdsourcing and Human Computation*, CHI

ACM, Vancouver, BC. Available at: http://crowdresearch.org/chi2011-workshop/ (accessed 26 September 2014).

Bohbot, V. D., McKenzie, S., Konishi, K., Fouquet, C., Kurdi, V., Schachar, R., and Robaey, P. (2012). Virtual Navigation Strategies from Childhood to Senescence: Evidence for Changes across the Life Span. *Frontiers in Aging Neuroscience*, 4: 28.

Bremmer, J. G. (1978). Egocentric Versus Allocentric Spatial Coding in Nine-month-old Infants: Factors Influencing the Choice of Code. *Developmental Psychology*, 14(4): 346–55.

Brown, P., Harniss, M., and Dudgeon, B. (2005). Barriers to Independence and Use of Technology. Paper presented at the *Alliance for Full Participation Summit*, September, Washington, DC.

Chan, E., Baumann, O., Bellgrove, M. A., and Mattingley, J. B. (2012). From Objects to Landmarks: The Function of Visual Location Information in Spatial Navigation. *Frontiers in Psychology*, 3: 304.

Chang, Y. -J. and Wang, T. -Y. (2010a). Comparing Picture and Video Prompting in Autonomous Indoor Wayfinding for Individuals with Cognitive Impairments. *Personal and Ubiquitous Computing*, 14(8): 737–47.

Chang, Y. -J. and Wang, T. -Y. (2010b). Indoor Wayfinding Based on Wireless Sensor Networks for Individuals with Multiple Special Needs. *Cybernetics and Systems*, 41(4): 317–33.

Chrastil, E. R. (2013). Neural Evidence Supports a Novel Framework for Spatial Navigation. *Psychonomic Bulletin and Review*, 20(2): 208–27.

Chu, Y., Brown, P., Harniss, M., Kautz, H., and Johnson, K. (2013). Cognitive Support Technologies for People with TBI: Current Usage and Challenges Experienced. *Disability Rehabilitation: Assistive Technology*, 9(4): 279–85.

Cicerone, K. D., Dahlberg, C., Kalmar, K., Langenbahn, D. M., Malec, J. F., and Berquist, T. F. (2000). Evidence-Based Cognitive Rehabilitation: Recommendations for Clinical Practice. *Archives of Physical Medicine and Rehabilitation*, 81(12): 1596–615.

Cook, A. M. and Polgar, J. M. (2007). *Cook and Hussey's Assistive Technologies: Principles and Practice*. St Louis, MO: Mosby Elsevier.

Courbois, Y., Blades, M., Farran, E. K., and Sockeel, P. (2013a). Do Individuals with Intellectual Disability Select Appropriate Objects as Landmarks when Learning a New Route? *Journal of Intellectual Disability Research*, 57(1): 80–9.

Courbois, Y., Farran, E. K., Lemahieu, A., Blades, M., Mengue-Topio, H., and Sockeel, P. (2013b). Wayfinding Behaviour in Down Syndrome: A Study with Virtual Environments. *Research on Developmental Disabilities*, 34(5): 1825–31.

de Joode, E. A., van Heugten, C., Verhey, F., and van Boxtel, M. (2010). Efficacy and Usability of Assistive Technology for Patients with Cognitive Deficits: A Systematic Review. *Clinical Rehabilitation*, 24: 701–14.

de Joode, E. A., van Boxtel, M. P. J., Verhey, F. R., and van Heugten, C. M. (2012). Use of Assistive Technology in Cognitive Rehabilitation: Exploratory Studies of the Opinions and Expectations of Healthcare Professionals and Potential Users. *Brain Injury*, 26(10): 1257–66.

Deipolyi, A. R., Rankin, K. P., Mucke, L., Miller, B. L., and Gorno-Tempini, M. L. (2007). Spatial Cognition and the Human Navigation Network in AD and MCI. *Neurology*, 69(10): 986–97.

Fallah, N., Apostolopoulos, I., Bekris, K., and Folmer, E. (2013). Indoor Human Navigation Systems: A Survey. *Interacting with Computers*, 25(1): 21–33.

Farran, E. K., Courbois, Y., Van Herwegen, J., and Blades, M. (2012). How Useful are Landmarks when Learning a Route in a Virtual Environment? Evidence from Typical Development and Williams' Syndrome. *Journal of Experimental Child Psychology*, 111(4): 571–86.

Fong, T., Finlayson, M., and Peacock, N. (2006). The Social Experience of Aging with a Chronic Illness: Perspectives of Older Adults with Multiple Sclerosis. *Disability and Rehabilitation*, 28(11): 695–705.

Frankenstein, J., Brussow, S., Ruzzoli, F., and Holscher, C. (2012). The Language of Landmarks: The Role of Background Knowledge in Indoor Wayfinding. *Cognitive Processing*, 13(1): S165–70.

Gillespie, A., Best, C., and O'Neill, B. (2011). Cognitive Function and Assistive Technology for Cognition: A Systematic Review. *Journal of the International Neuropsychological Society*, 18(1): 1.

Hart, T., O'Neil-Pirozzi, T., and Morita, C. (2003). Clinician Expectations for Portable Electronic Devices as Cognitive-Behavioural Orthoses in Traumatic Brain Injury Rehabilitation. *Brain Injury*, 17(5): 401–11.

Head, D. and Isom, M. (2010). Age Effects on Wayfinding and Route Learning Skills. *Behavioural Brain Research*, 209(1): 49–58.

Iaria, G., Palermo, L., Committeri, G., and Barton, J. J. (2009). Age Differences in the Formation and use of Cognitive Maps. *Behavioural Brain Research*, 196(2): 187–91.

Kettunen, P., Irvankoski, K., Krause, C. M., and Sarjakoski, L. T. (2013). Landmarks in Nature to Support Wayfinding: The Effects of Seasons and Experimental Methods. *Cognitive Processes*, 14(3): 245–53.

Kirsch, N. L., Shenton, M., Spirl, E., Rowan, J., Simpson, R., Schreckenghost, D., and LoPresti, E. F. (2004). Web-Based Assistive Technology Interventions for Cognitive Impairments After Traumatic Brain Injury: A Selective Review and Two Case Studies. *Rehabilitation Psychology*, 49(3): 200–12.

Klatzky, R. L. (1998). Allocentric and Egocentric Spatial Representations: Definitions, Distinctions and Interconnections. In Freksa, C., Habel, C., and Wender, K. F. (eds), *Spatial Cognition: An Interdisciplinary Approach to Representing and Processing Spatial Knowledge* (pp. 1–17). Berlin, Germany: Springer-Verlag.

Lancioni, G. E., O'Reilly, M. F., Singh, N. N., Sigafoos, J., and Oliva, D. (2009). Orientation Technology for Indoor Travel by Persons with Multiple Disabilities. *Cognitive Processes*, 10(2): 244–6.

Lehnung, M., Leplow, B., Friege, L., Herzog, A., and Ferstl, R. (1998). Development of Spatial Memory and Spatial Orientation in Preschoolers and Primary School Children. *British Journal of Psychology*, 89: 463–80.

Lemoncello, R., Sohlberg, M. M., and Fickas, S. (2010). When Directions Fail: Investigation of Getting Lost Behaviour in Adults with Acquired Brain Injury. *Brain Injury*, 24(3): 550–9.

Liao, L., Patterson, D. J., Fox, D., and Kautz, H. (2007). Learning and Inferring Transportation Routines. *Artificial Intelligence*, 171: 311–31.

Lind, S. E., Williams, D. M., Raber, J., Peel, A., and Bowler, D. M. (2013). Spatial Navigation Impairments among Intellectually High-Functioning Adults with Autism Spectrum Disorder: Exploring Relations with Theory of Mind, Episodic Memory, and Episodic Future Thinking. *Journal of Abnormal Psychology*, 122(4): 1189–99.

Litvak, S. and Enders, A. (2001). Support Systems: The Interface Between Individuals and Environments (pp. 711–33). In Albrecht, G. L., Seelman, K., and Bury, M. (eds), *Handbook of Disability Studies*. Thousand Oaks, CA: Sage.

Liu, A. L. (2010). *Design of an Adaptive Wayfinding System for Individuals with Cognitive Impairments* (PhD). Seattle: University of Washington.

Liu, A. L., Hile, H., Borriello, G., Kautz, H., Ferris, B., Brown, P. A., and Johnson, K. (2006). Implications for Location Systems in Indoor Wayfinding for Individuals with Cognitive Impairments (pp. 1–5). In *Proceedings of the Pervasive Health Conference and Workshops*, November 29–December 1, Innsbruck. doi: 10.1109/PCTHEALTH.2006.361699.

Liu, A. L., Hile, H., Kautz, H., Borriello, G., Brown, P. A., Harniss, M., and Johnson, K. (2008). Indoor Wayfinding: Developing a Functional Interface for Individuals with Cognitive Impairments. *Disability and Rehabilitation: Assistive Technology*, 3(1): 69–81.

Liu, A. L., Hile, H., Borriello, G., Kautz, H., Brown, P., Harniss, M., and Johnson, K. (2009). Informing the Design of an Automated Wayfinding System for Individuals with Cognitive Impairments (pp. 1–8). In *Proceedings of the International Conference on Pervasive Computing Technologies for Healthcare*, London. doi: 10.4108/ICST. PERVASIVEHEALTH2009.6018.

Liu, A. L., Borriello, G., Kautz, H., Brown, P. A., Harniss, M., and Johnson, K. (2010). Learning User Models to Improve Wayfinding Assistance for Individuals with Cognitive Impairment (pp. 105–8). In *Proceedings of the First International Workshop on Interactive Systems in Healthcare*, April 1–3, Atlanta, GA.

Mengue-Topio, H., Courbois, Y., Farran, E. K., and Sockeel, P. (2011). Route Learning and Shortcut Performance in Adults with Intellectual Disability: A Study with Virtual Environments. *Research in Developmental Disabilities*, 32(1): 345–52.

Overman, W. H., Pate, B. J., Moore, K., and Peuster, A. (1996). Ontogeny of Place Learning in Children as Measured in the Radial Arm Maze, Morris Search Task and Open Field Task. *Behavioral Neuroscience*, 110: 1205–28.

Paas, F., Renkl, A., and Sweller, J. (2003). Cognitive Load Theory and Instructional Design: Recent Developments. *Educational Psychologist*, 38(1): 1–4.

Piajet, J. and Inhelder, B. (1948). *The Child's Conception of Space*. New York, NY: Norton.

Scherer, M. J. and Craddock, G. (2002). Matching Person and Technology (MPT) Assessment Process. *Technology and Disability*, 14(3): 125–31.

Scottish Intercollegiate Guidelines Network. (2008). *SIGN 50: A Guideline Developer's Handbook*. Edinburgh: Scottish Intercollegiate Guidelines Network.

Siegel, A. W. and White, S. H. (1975). The Development of Spatial Representations of Large Environments. *Advances in Child Development and Behavior* (pp. 9–55). New York, NY: Academic Press.

Sohlberg, M., Fickas, S., Hung, P., and Fortier, A. (2007). A Comparison of Four Prompt Modes for Route Finding for Community Travellers with Severe Cognitive Impairments. *Brain Injury*, 21(5): 531–8.

Speake, J. and Axon, S. (2012). "I Never Use 'Maps' Anymore": engaging with Satnav Technologies and the Implications for Cartographic Literacy and Spatial Awareness. *The Cartographic Journal*, (e-pub July 26), 49(4): 326–36.

Stephenson, J. and Limbrick, L. (2013). A Review of the use of Touch-Screen Mobile Devices by People with Developmental Disabilities. *Journal of Autism and Developmental Disorders*. doi: 10.1007/s10803-013-1878-8.

US Census Bureau (2014). *American Fact Finder*. Available at: http://factfinder2.census.gov (accessed 11 June 2014).

Uc, E. Y., Rizzo, M., Anderson, S. W., Sparks, J. D., Rodnitzky, R. L., and Dawson, J. D. (2007). Impaired Navigation in Drivers with Parkinson's Disease. *Brain*, 130(9): 2433–40.

van der Ham, I. J., Kant, N., Postma, A., and Visser-Meily, J. M. (2013). Is Navigation Ability a Problem in Mild Stroke Patients? Insights from Self-Reported Navigation Measures. *Journal of Rehabilitation Medicine*, 45(5): 429–33.

Wiedenbauer, G. and Jansen-Osmann, P. (2006). Spatial Knowledge of Children with Spina Bifida in a Virtual Large-Scale Space. *Brain and Cognition*, 62(2): 120–7.

Wiener, J. M., Büchner, S. J., and Hölscher, C. (2009). Taxonomy of Human Wayfinding Tasks: A Knowledge-Based Approach. *Spatial Cognition and Computation*, 9(2): 152–65.

Woollett, K. and Maguire, E. A. (2010). The Effect of Navigational Expertise on Wayfinding in New Environments. *Journal of Environmental Psychology*, 30(4–2): 565–73.

11

THE FUTURE OF ASSISTIVE TECHNOLOGY FOR COGNITION

Alex Gillespie and Brian O'Neill

In chapter one, we proposed a model of cognition as distributed in a functional loop which includes the brain, other people, and technologies. Over the past 150 years we have made strides in understanding the neural element in cognition and action. We can assert, with confidence, that human cognition is grounded in the neural architecture of the human brain. But we can also be confident that a full understanding of human cognition, as it occurs in daily living, must consider elements beyond the brain itself; namely, the social and technical milieu within which that neural structure is embedded (Hutchins, 1995).

To conceptualize the distributed nature of cognitive function we returned to Bateson (1972: 465) and the idea of "total circuits." He did not see the brain level, person level or technology level in isolation as sufficient to describe cognition. Rather, he conceptualized cognition in functional terms as a property of the whole circuit; that is, the set of inter-relations between the person, the social world, and the technology. Thus, for example, an explanation for behavior will likely entail representations, which are distributed between the individual, the environment, tools, and even, in the cases of joint activity, other people (Norman, 2002; Tomasello *et al.*, 2005; see also Alm, Chapter 7 of this volume).

Development of the cognitive function is dependent on the scaffolds that people and environments provide (Vygotsky, 1997; Pea, 2004; see also Räsänen *et al.*, Chapter 8 of this volume). Similarly, in decline or illness, those supports in the environment again become critical (Baltes, 1997). Damage to the brain leads to impairment, and it is common for caregivers to become assistants for cognition, reminding, directing, prompting, and guiding the individual (O'Neill and Gillespie, 2008). The developments of technologies that augment the cognitive processes have huge potential to restore function, but implementation is challenging. These technologies need accessible interfaces, they need to be supported by the social milieu, and they need to respond to the genuine interests of people with cognitive impairment. Technologies cannot be seen as assisting cognition in isolation; rather, they need to be conceptualized within the full neuro-socio-technical loop.

To conceptualize the "neuro" segment of the neuro-socio-technical model we employed the International Classification of Function (ICF, World Health Organization (WHO), 2002), and specifically the categorization of Specific Mental Functions. For each of the cognitive functions in the ICF, we sought out experts who could review and present the state-of-the-art ATC for the given functional domain. Our chapters subsumed the ICF specific mental functions (with ICF chapter number) as follows:

Chapter 2, *Assistive technology for arousal, alertness*, and *attention*, addressed *attention functions* (b140) and the authors demonstrated technologies that aid *concentration*, *sustaining attention*, and *shifting attention*. The authors did not find supports for *divided attention* or *sharing attention*.

Chapter 3, *Assistive technology for memory*, dealt with the *memory functions* (b144). This chapter presented supports for *retrieval of memory* (b1442) and *long-term memory* (b1441), but not *short-term memory* (b1440), defined as a "temporary, disruptable memory store of around 30 seconds duration from which information is lost if not consolidated into long-term memory" (WHO, 2002).

Chapter 4, *Affect-aware assistive technologies*, addressed emotional functions (b152). This chapter presented evidence that current technologies can use a variety of methods to sense and feedback on the *range of emotions* (b1522), that we are at the beginning of development of technologies to help with *regulation of emotion* (b1521), and, in the case of face recognition and feedback to people with autistic spectrum disorders, that we may be able to support *appropriateness of emotion* (b1520).

Chapter 5, *Assistive technology for disorders of visual perception*, dealt with *perceptual functions* (b156). The authors specifically addressed *visual perception* (b1561) and *visuospatial perception* (b1565). The chapter necessarily omitted supports for *auditory perception* (b1560), *olfactory perception* (b1562), *gustatory perception* (b1563), and *tactile perception* (b1564).

Chapter 6, *Assistive technology for executive functions*, surveyed supports for the *higher-level cognitive functions* (b164), demonstrating technologies to support *organization and planning* (b1641) and *time management* (b1642). The chapter authors did not find assistive technology to support *abstraction* (b1640), *cognitive flexibility* (b1643), *insight* (b1644), *judgment* (b1645), and *problem solving* (b1646), and so the development of real-time supports for such functions remain challenging and tantalizing goals for the field.

Chapter 7, *Cognitive support for language and social interaction*, addressed *mental functions of language* (b167). The well-developed field of augmentative and assistive communication has created technologies to support *expression of language* (b1671), *integrative language functions* (b1672; those "mental functions that organize semantic and symbolic meaning, grammatical structure, and ideas for the production of messages in spoken, written or other forms of language") and, to an extent, *reception of language* (b1670). It begged the question as to whether technologies that change the speed of incoming messages or allow replay might be clinically useful in this area.

Chapter 8, *Assistive technology for supporting learning numeracy*, addressed calculation functions (b172); "the specific Assistive Technology for Supporting Learning Numeracy mental functions of determination, approximation, and manipulation of mathematical symbols and processes, focusing on supports which adapt to user performance to maximally enable their ability" (WHO, 2002).

Chapter 9, *Assistive technology for psychomotor functioning and sequencing complex movements*, subsumed both mental function of *sequencing complex movements* (b176; mental functions of sequencing and coordinating complex, purposeful movements) and *psychomotor functions* (b147; mental functions of control over both motor and psychological events at the body level). The authors persuasively demonstrated that computer vision can enable awareness of movement patterns so that support can be given when needed. The success of clinical applications in select groups (people with dementia) invites recruitment of other clinical groups.

Chapter 10, *Cognitive technologies for wayfinding*, addressed aspects of *experience of self and time functions* (b180; namely, *awareness of one's position in the reality of one's environment and of time*) though necessarily omitted awareness of one's identity body (albeit Chapter 2 does cover some aspects of improving attention to neglected body areas).

Overall, the ICF worked well as a framework to conceptualize the neuro component of the neuro-socio-technical circuit, and we have been able to map specific social activities and technical devices onto most of the ICF categories. We did have trouble finding authors to specifically address the ICF categories *experience of self and time* (b180) and *thought functions* (b160). Technologies for experience of self and time were found to be rare, and, thus, insufficient to form a stand-alone chapter. The few ATC that do augment this cognitive function were, to some extent, in Chapter 10 on navigation. The ICF category "thought functions" is very broad, and, again, it was difficult to find relevant ATC. It is difficult to both assess and augment phenomena such as pressure of thought, flight of ideas, thought block, incoherence of thought, tangentiality, circumstantiality, delusions, obsessions and compulsions, as well as de-realization from current reality.

The fact that ATC only augments a limited subset of the cognitive functions offers a challenge to neuropsychologists and technologists to develop ATC to address the functions thus far neglected. Accordingly, a secondary contribution of using the ICF has been to identify the cognitive functions for which technological assistance is lacking and, thus, which might have potential for future research. To begin this process, this chapter will review some potentially useful lines for development for future ATC and also consider some of the challenges facing ATC as it moves into the future.

Predicting the future: a note of caution

Making future predictions is an activity that most academics are wise enough to avoid. The history of such predictions contains more error than accuracy. Predictions about the future age poorly, usually appearing as a peculiar product of their time. Looking back over predictions about the future, two things are evident: first, that predictions are biased toward what currently exists, extrapolating from the present; for example, that there will be more of the same, but it will be smaller, cheaper, faster, better, and so on. This is likely because thinking about the future activates areas of the brain associated with memories of what has been (Schacter *et al.*, 2008). The paradigm shifts, the genuine innovations, and the surprises, are invariably omitted (Taleb, 2010). For example, very few predictions over the last hundred years foresaw the digital revolution, the Internet or the mobile phone – yet, most predictions included faster trains and cars. The mobility of phones is a key case to reveal the conceptual leaps required for prediction. Telephony has had patent protection since 1876 and the first commercially available mobile phone appeared in 1983; yet, the idea of cellular mobile telephony was proposed only in 1947 (Ring, 1947). Second, there seems to be a tendency toward both unrealistic optimism (Weinstein, 1982) and what is called *immune neglect* (Gilbert *et al.*, 1998), which is the tendency to catastrophize negative predictions, failing to take account of how well we cope with adversity. Taken together, these two tendencies mean that our predictions about the future tend to be much more exciting than the future usually turns out to be.

Given such slim chances of success, why take the risk of predicting the future of ATC? Humans are future-oriented and goal-directed (Karniol and Ross, 1996). It is, therefore, part of the human predicament that we cannot predict the future, but we are condemned to be guided by our predictions. We act with purpose, oriented to a future, yet, the historical record shows that unintended consequences are common (Merton, 1936). Avoidance of prediction may be wise for those reluctant to be wrong. But, avoidance would have us give up important questions simply because they are difficult.

Already, bold thinking by clinicians and technologists about the potentials of technology has led to breakthroughs. Based on achievements in the description of cognitive function, the technologies AbleLink, Affectiva, Alertness Cushion, AmbienNet, aQRdate, Archipel, AssistMote, Autominder, Biofeedback, Calcularis, CHAT, CIRCA, COGORTH, COACH, Content free cuing, Contralesional Neck Vibration, Disease Management Assistance System, Emotional Hearing Aid, Fresnel Prism Glasses, Gestele, Google Glass, Guide, ICue, Intelligent Wheelchairs, Kinept, Limb Activation Device, Lingraphica, Locompt, LookTel, Memex, MemoJOG, MIT Manus, Neure, NeuroPage, NoiseCancellingHeadphones, NumberRace, Opportunity Knocks, PEAT, Psion organizer, Q-Sensor, Real Directions, SelfCam, SenseCam, Social Robots, Sonic Guide, Standup, TalksBack, TapTapSee, Television Assisted Prompting, TextDetective, Transcranial magnetic and direct current stimulation, VibroGlove, VizWiz, and Watchminder are all intellectual contributions which envisaged how that cognitive function might be augmented; they were bold strides into the future. Accordingly, with an awareness of our limited capacity for forecasting and inspiration from those who have already instituted novel ATC, we proceed to offer the following speculations.

Future potentials

It seems highly likely that the digital revolution will continue apace, with improvements in components, personalization, and interfaces. First, regarding components, computing power and data storage will become cheaper and increasingly mobile. The cost and quality of sensors will continue to improve, and new sensors will be developed. These factors will lead to a surge in wearable computing (smartphones, smart glasses, smart watches; smart clothes and smart technologies that we might assimilate and *wear* within our bodies) and ubiquitous computing (smart appliances, smart homes, and smart environments).

Second, the improvement and spread of components will feed into increased personalization. Wearable and ubiquitous computing is already leading to massive data collection on users, and increasingly this data will allow software to be tailored to the user. Central to personalization is having data on the user, such as previous activities, performance, social encounters, purchasing choices, journeys, and preferences. This "big data" does not homogenize individuals, but rather particularizes them, enabling smart devices to tailor services to the individual. This already occurs when an Internet search engine takes account of the user's location or previous search history to tailor results. In this way ATC will become more contextual (see Manly and O'Neill, Chapter 2 of this volume), more aware of what is going on and of what the user is trying to achieve, and thus less "dumb." Past behavior predicts future behavior, and a technology with awareness of past patterns might be used to make suggestions when these do not come to mind and then help support achievement of those goals.

Third, it is likely that the way in which we interact with ATC will change hugely. Until recently, interfaces allowed manual input (keyboards and mice) and visual feedback (screens). Recently, touchscreen, gestural recognition, and natural language interfaces have become common. Augmented vision is set to become more widespread. For example, Google Glass, mentioned in Chapters 2, 6, and 9, seems like a promising new platform. Although it does not yet provide augmented vision, it is possible that future versions will. Also, it is just one of several similar interfaces being developed, such as by Samsung, Optinvent, ChipSiP, Epson, and Vuzix, and these alternatives will have somewhat different characteristics (e.g. bigger screens, more or less augmented reality, different software). Moreover, technologists are also exploring radically different interfaces, which break away from the tendency toward visual interfaces. For example, companies such as InteraXon and Advanced Brain Monitoring have mobile multi-channel EEG monitoring systems that relay data in real time to a smartphone, which, in turn, can either store the data or send an alert. Might EEG or other mobile brain monitoring equipment be used to interact with ATC? At the most extreme end of this trend are explorations in "wet" interfaces, where the technology directly interacts with the users nervous system (Hochberg et al., 2012).

Considering these three broad trends, alongside the chapters in the present volume, lead us to speculate that near future ATC advances will focus on: (1) recognizing objects, actions, emotions, and faces, (2) emotion regulation, (3) executive function, (4) everyday life navigation.

Recognizing objects, actions, faces, and emotions

There is a lot of interest in being able to search images and videos on the Internet. While text search has progressed hugely, the massive data pile of images and videos on the Internet has remained more difficult to search. Accordingly, a lot of resources are being put into developing algorithms which will be able to search multimedia data to find objects, landmarks, faces, spoken phrases, actions (Pirsiavash and Ramanan, 2012), and even emotions (e.g. software by Emotient and Realeyes). These algorithms will likely have many secondary functions, such as making robots more intelligent. We also expect that they will be used to power novel ATC.

First, inability to recognize objects, faces, emotions, and actions can cause significant disability. Simply using these new algorithms to inform users could have a significant beneficial impact (who would not like a device that puts names to the faces of distant acquaintances). One can imagine recognition occurring in real time and users informed via devices such as Google Glass, or the forthcoming equivalents from Samsung, Optinvent, ChipSiP, Epson, and Vuzix, providing discrete visual or audio recognition functionality. Or, maybe, the information will be provided by an augmented visual overlay, smartphone, smart watch, or some other platform. One could also imagine such algorithms being paired with mobile eyetracking solutions (e.g. as are being developed by SensoMotoric Instruments), such that whatever the user looks at (whether it is an object, landmark, or face) leads the system to make an identification and then feed the name or relevant information back to the user through various channels.

Second, these recognition algorithms will likely be used in more complex prompting and planning ATC because they will enable more contextually relevant prompts. Guide (O'Neill et al., 2010), for example, has no capacity for monitoring users' activities except by asking the user to report what stage of the activity they are at. COACH, however, does have an artificial intelligence component that attempts to infer the stage of activity from video data (Mihailidis et al., 2011). Both of these devices would benefit from powerful algorithms for real-time recognizing people, objects, and activities in video data.

A potential third consequence of these algorithms for recognition is that the data can be manipulated before being fed back to the user. For example, words can be translated into a different language (e.g. Microsoft's simultaneous verbal translation for Skype), or associations can be made to the data based on the semantic web in general, or personalized data based on the user. Thus, not only would a user obtain the name for the face, but also information about previous interactions, relevant emails, future meetings with the person which are in a calendar, and so on. The system might even suggest suitable conversation openings or provide reminders to ask the identified person about some relevant information.

Emotion regulation

The recognition systems mentioned above can be used to recognize emotional states in other people, but it is also possible to use technology to recognize emotional states in the user. Feeding back to users their own emotional state may be able to support emotion regulation. Emotional dysregulation is a prominent feature of many disorders of brain function. This neurobehavioral disability (Wood, 2001) is causative in relationship and social functioning difficulties (Bond *et al.*, 1979), and contributes to relationship instability and the burden of care (Gosling and Oddy, 1999). Through the inseparable nature of emotional response and cognition, emotional dysregulation also contributes to disabling impairments of judgment and problem solution (Bechara *et al.*, 1997).

Technologies that can sense, process, and feedback on current emotional state promise a revolution in the treatment of emotional dysregulation. Current management is divisible into three broad categories: *medical*, attempting to address the physiological dysfunction; *psychological*, changing behavioral or cognitive activity to alter emotional state; and *containment* of those with severe emotional dysregulation to manage the risks posed. The medical approach to emotional dysregulation offers some options with a gradually increasing evidence base (Fleminger *et al.*, 2006). The psychological approaches are exemplified in neurobehavioral rehabilitation, where specially trained staff in the milieu provide feedback on emotional and behavioral states with the effect of reducing the frequency and intensity of behaviors reflecting emotional dysregulation (Worthington *et al.*, 2006; Oddy and da Silva Ramos, 2013). Thus, by increasing awareness of emotional state, in self and others, the person can better regulate their emotional expression. The key to this long-term rehabilitative effect is the feedback to the service user as to the effect of their behavior on others, with the aim of bringing about greater alignment in the emotional states of the persons interacting (Bowen *et al.*, 2010). Devices that can function as tools in this feedback process will be an important fourth class of tools in addressing emotional and behavioral dysregulation.

Specifically, emotion regulation ATC will likely use multiple channels of monitoring, including physiological indicators (i.e. GSR, heart rate, agitation of movement) and information about location, co-present people, and activities, to assess changes in emotional state. This information could then be fed back to the user (again via discrete audio or visual display, or, in this case, maybe haptic feedback, such as a vibration alert, would be suitable). If the situation escalated it might also be appropriate to feed the warning indicators to caregivers or clinical staff who would be able to intervene before severe emotional escalation occurs.

Executive function

Executive function likely occupies the greatest amount of neural territory (Burgess *et al.*, 2011) and is one of the areas of cognitive function wherein we are currently making the greatest inroads. The ICF posits that the higher-order cognitive function processes (executive functions) include: abstraction from events; organization, planning, executing actions; time management; cognitive flexibility; insight; judgment. According to our assessment, we have so far developed supports for organization, planning, executing actions, and time management. Thus, there remain a lot of thought functions that have yet to be assisted by technology. We see potential for future ATC to augment working memory, judgment, and general problem solving.

Working memory function has been associated with a wide range of positive outcomes (Alloway and Alloway, 2010). It is an elementary task for technology to record information in real time. Accordingly, if there were some way to enable people to interrogate the previous 30 seconds or so of real-time recording rapidly and efficiently, then it might be possible to have an augmentation of working memory. The design challenge is not so much in maintaining a recording of the previous 30 seconds, but in making that data accessible to cognitive operations in real time. An example illustrating the potential of this idea is the Conversation Prompter (Orpwood *et al.*, 2007). Again, the platform for such an interface might be a new wearable computer, such as a visual display worn on glasses, or an in-ear augmentation (e.g. Dash smart ear buds) or, indeed, an as yet unrealized potential for easy mobile direct brain stimulation.

Augmenting general problem solving might also be possible. One could imagine a verbal or visual interface that supports users in thinking through a problem, scaffolding the user in thinking through the major steps in generic problem solving. For example, the system would encourage the user to identify problems, specify their goals, work out the actions necessary for each goal, identify necessary resources, and determine which actions are most likely to succeed. It might even be that simply encouraging people to talk aloud (Ericsson and Simon, 1993; Wagoner and Gillespie, 2014) and then having that talk played back to the user enables them to better reflect upon their own thought processes, potentially identifying their own biases or unrealistic cognitions. One could also imagine how judgment and self-regulation could be augmented within such a system, as the system monitors activities and checks them against goals. For example, the system might prompt self-reflection or self-regulation by asking "what is your priority now?" or even just reminding users of their previously defined priorities.

Everyday life navigation

Devices that provide navigation prompts based on GPS data have revolutionized road navigation for drivers. There is a lot of potential for further refining this basic form of technological assistance (Boger *et al.*, 2014). First, in the near future, it is likely that positioning data will be both more accurate and also work indoors. Knowing a user's precise location and orientation, and the history of both, can inform several ATC; for example, leading to more contextual prompts. Second, it is likely that this information will be increasingly linked to datasets, such as the user's calendar, their to-do list, and their communications, and also more general databases about transport, events, landmarks, news, and tasks. Thus, the spatial navigation ATC of the future will likely not only tell a user when to turn left or right, but also where and when to buy a ticket, when and where to get some lunch while waiting for the ticket queue to reduce; or, maybe the system will bypass the queue altogether, and manage to book the ticket online for the user. But the point is that "spatial navigation" will move into "social space navigation" or "everyday life navigation;" that is, guiding users not only through geographic space but also through social activities. For example, if the user's plane is delayed, the system will not only notify them, but also suggest hotels, nearby eateries, and interesting landmarks. Such a device could also be linked to social networking, so that the user is informed about nearby acquaintances, or acquaintances of acquaintances with whom a common interest is shared, and so on. Thus, we anticipate a greater merger between spatial navigation devices and prompting devices.

Future challenges

The future of ATC will not be determined solely by technological advances, but it will also be shaped by user desires and, especially, resistance to use (Bauer, 2014). ATC which are cumbersome to use or have the unintended consequence of making disabilities publicly visible, or technologies which are intrusive or enable undesirable surveillance are likely to be resisted by users (see also Jamieson and Evans, Chapter 6 of this volume). In short, to reduce resistance, future ATC should focus less on the regulation of people with cognitive impairments as upon enabling people to achieve their own goals.

Empowering users

Information flow will be a key factor in the neuro-socio-technical model. A large number of technologies are basically communication technologies, usually sending messages to remind or prompt the user. These information flows can be directed in several ways, to others, such as caregivers, or looping back to the user. The former can be labeled negatively, with terms like tagging, monitoring or spying. The latter, feedback, philosophically sits more comfortably with most as it augments the natural capacities of the individual through knowledge. The feedback loop is critically important in most forms of cognition; trial and error and trial and success are those processes by which we hone our skilled action. But we see both feedback and "feed out" as necessary to optimize autonomous action fully. Service users will require to consent to the service, to receive and share information. Those accessing the information will require to consent to use that information only in the service of the user.

Accordingly, we propose that an important conceptual distinction to make with ATC is who is in control of the device, and specifically whether the control is external or internal to the user (Best *et al.*, 2014). Indeed, arguably, as control becomes more external, then the device becomes less of an ATC and more of a means of controlling someone. For example, a smart-home system, which monitors the occupant by sending a notification to a caregiver if a certain profile of behavior is matched, provides external control. However, a smart-home system, which monitors the occupant and sends the occupant a notification when the same profile is matched, is cultivating the awareness of the occupant, scaffolding and supporting the occupant to monitor their own behavior. In this sense, all ATC that encourage internal control might be seen to support attention also, encouraging the user to monitor their mood, the time, their diary, other people, steps in a task or whatever (see O'Neill and Manly, Chapter 2 of this volume). Whether future ATC work with users' cognitive functions or supplant them is not merely a clinical decision, it is also a decision with ethical implications that users may well have opinions about (Wherton and Monk, 2008). From a social psychological point of view, we suspect that the more future ATC supports internal control, the more users will attribute improved functioning to their own agency, rather than the technology, and thus the less the resistance to adopting the technology.

Supporting users' identity

Dependence on others for activities of daily living is rarely desirable; it can lead to stigma (Goffman, 1963) and a spoiled identity within close relationships (Gillespie *et al.*, 2010). Maintenance of acquired skills for as long as possible is a stated aim of most people with disabilities (Baltes, 1997). While restoring abilities has obvious practical benefits, it also supports the user's identity by repositioning the person within social relations. Rather than relationships being characterized by dependency, they are more likely to be characterized by equality. ATC that support users to have positive identities will likely be adopted. What evidence is there for ATC working with, rather than against, users' identities?

Prompting technologies addressed by Jamieson and Evans (see Chapter 6 of this volume), Dewar, Kopelman, Kapur, and Wilson (see Chapter 3), and Boger and Mihailidis (see Chapter 9) allow a person to take agency for achievement of set behaviors and sequences of behavior. Independence of activity serves to reposition a person from cared-for to becoming an equal partner in the relationship. In the case of scaffolding activities of daily living, such as the making of food and drinks, people move from the position of being in receipt of kindness to being able to offer kindness once again (e.g. being able to offer someone a cup of tea).

AlZoubi, Hussain, and Calvo, in their chapter on emotion (see Chapter 4), demonstrate that those perhaps most marginalized by specific impairment, those with autistic spectrum disorders, may be supported to recognize the emotional state of others, may receive support in regulating their emotion in difficult social situations, and may receive reminder prompts as to how to get by in a social situation. Combined, these could have massive benefits in repositioning. Robertson and colleagues, whose work was described in the chapter on attention (see O'Neill and Manly, Chapter 2), reported evidence that biofeedback to increase arousal led to reports of greater social involvement, that by energizing people they utilized this activation to seek out social interaction.

Fostering receptive social environments

In addition to ATC being useful and non-stigmatizing to the user, they also need to be supported by the cultural norms and attitudes of significant others. The decision to engage in any one behavior, including technology use, is influenced by the person's attitude to that behavior and the subjective norm, the course which the person believes others would have them follow (Ajzen and Fishbein, 1980; Fishbein and Ajzen, 1975), and the perceived ability to carry out that behavior (Ajzen, 1991). This theory may be drawn into our model. The use of any one assistive technology is influenced by *attitude*, which may in turn be impacted by device aesthetics, ergonomics, and emotional factors; *subjective norm*, which will be influenced by evidence of efficacy, media portrayal, and vicarious experience; and *perceived behavioral control*, which will be influenced by cognitive factors, experience, and effort to use. Thus, future ATC should be considered not only in relation to the individual user, but also in relation to the user's social network and how that network will support, or resist, the new technology.

Creating interfaces tailored to cognitive profiles

A fourth aspect to user adoption is the cognitive demands of using the ATC. For example, Jamieson and Evans (see Chapter 9) make the interesting point that, despite evidence for ATC for executive function, there has been relatively little uptake. They point to the particularly difficult problem that using contemporary ATC often requires a substantial degree of cognitive function. Thus, they argue, there needs to be more research on matching interfaces with cognitive profiles. As Harniss, Brown, and Johnson point out (see Chapter 10), similar personalization is necessary to make wayfinding devices accessible. Research, accordingly, should focus not only on identifying which ATC ameliorate which impairments, but also which interfaces are most adapted to which impairments.

One consideration that moderates the concern about complex interfaces is that people themselves are adapting to new technology and, as such, what seems like a complex interface today may seem routine and familiar in a decade. The cognitive component of the neuro-socio-technical loop adapts to the technological component. Cognition is different when it is unaided compared with when it is supported by pen and paper or a word processor, which allows for ideas to be remembered, sorted, and refined (Heim, 1999). Indeed, there is already evidence that people's cognitive processes have adapted to Internet search (Carr, 2010). The key point here is that, in speculating about the future of ATC, it is likely that issues which cause some user resistance today will simply fade out with time (and likely be replaced by new concerns).

Developing a policy framework for prescription

Identifying the most effective ATC for a given individual will require expert knowledge of the technologies available, the evidence base for efficacy and the given individual's cognitive profile. Neuropsychologists have this expertise and would be among the first to claim prescribing rights for ATC. There are many reasons why we would argue that ATC use might best be encouraged within a neuropsychological framework. First, an understanding of the functional impairments is required, both the cognitive functions and the activities of daily living which depend on them. Second, the efficacy evidence would need to be accessed, to prescribe for the known impairments in the light of the likely outcome. Third, there will be cognitive factors that need to be taken into account in technology use. In such a neuropsychological rehabilitation setting, awareness of deficit can be enhanced, clear goals set, service users trained in the use of devices (using techniques such as errorless learning to overcome memory impairments), devices trialed safely, effectiveness monitored, adjustment discussed, and generalization encouraged by gradually increasing the environments in which the function is exercised. Such support for users, we suspect, will be critical to ensuring that ATC is effective in real-world settings.

New assessments, new technologies, new learning, and efficacy analysis will require new services for the care of those with impairments. These will need to be service led, not technology led. The information on which the technologies run and support people in intimate areas of life will need to be handled sensitively, requiring reliable and secure data-processing infrastructures. Thus, we suggest that information and communication technologists may increasingly become members of the rehabilitation team.

Building the evidence base

There is increasing evidence for the efficacy of ATC in emotion regulation, experience of self in relation to place, and memory. The developments of computer systems, which closely emulate the cognitive functions of object, face, and voice recognition, object tracking, perception of facial emotion, lexical and word comprehension, semantic search, and complex problem solution, promise many more areas of cognitive support in the near future; but only if we have the paradigm shift we and authors have called for. The majority of these technologies, like the pocket calculator, though likely plausibly useful to us, have not been clinically tested.

In order to prescribe ATC there needs to be a robust evidence base. The current problem is that there are far more ATC devices than there are clinical trials. For example, facial recognition and object recognition are now possible, but we have not found any clinical trials using this technology with people who have a disability recognizing faces or objects. This lack of evidence is likely due to the number of devices, the cost of conducting proper trials, and the rapid development of the field. Given these reasons, it would be naïve to suggest only that more randomized control trials are required. Rather, what is needed is a strategic approach to randomized control trials that will enable generalization to a range of ATC devices.

Conceptualizing ATC in terms of the broad cognitive functions of alerting, directing attention, prompting, navigating, reminding, and storing and displaying (Gillespie *et al.*, 2012) enables generalization of research findings. This ICF classification enables generalization of specific ATC trial results toward general ATC functions. Given the proliferation of unique ATC devices, it is not practical to conduct large-scale studies of efficacy for each new device. For example, the robust RCT of NeuroPage (Wilson *et al.*, 2001) does more than suggest the efficacy of pagers, but rather demonstrates the basic finding that reminding ATC utilizing text or voice statements of the intended action reduce behavioral omissions. This same effect, it is reasonable to assume, could be achieved using an Android or iOS smartphone. Thus, the field needs to look beyond the specific hardware or software implementations, to see the underlying functionality being tested.

Conclusion

The evidence, as of 2014, allows a number of summary points (Gillespie *et al.*, 2012; Best *et al.*, 2013, 2014): first, the evidence base for ATC efficacy is growing rapidly. The preponderance of single case and small number studies echoes the early history of neuropsychology itself. Larger scale, randomized trials will be resource intensive, but the investments are likely to be recouped via technology provision and enablement-mediated care savings. Second, the focus has thus far been on reminding (especially prospective remembering and goal maintenance; see Jamieson and Evans, Chapter 6), prompting (see Boger and Mihailidis, Chapter 9), and alerting (see O'Neill and Manly, Chapter 2) devices. Nevertheless, ATC for other cognitive functions, such as storing and accessing information, navigating, emotion sensing, calculation, and perceiving, are growing.

While there may be a temptation to conceptualize ATC in terms of either technologies or disabilities, we argue that the most useful way forward is categorization by cognitive function. Technological categorizations are of limited use for prescribing because the same technological platform (e.g. a smartphone or head-mounted display) can be used for many different purposes. Classifying ATC in terms of diagnostic classes would obscure the functional cognitive impairments that are common to these conditions. For example, the devices covered in the preceding chapters can be used for attention deficit hyperactivity disorder, autistic spectrum disorders, Alzheimer's dementia, Asperger's syndrome, bipolar disorder, brain tumors, intellectual developmental disability, learning disability, Parkinson's, traumatic brain injury, schizophrenia, stroke, and vascular dementia, among others. Such diagnostic classes are useful for identifying the underlying cause of cognitive impairment, but they are less useful for implementing functional assistance because multiple causes can lead to the same functional deficit (e.g. planning deficits). Moreover, we are hopeful for cross-fertilization, where clinicians and developers working with a specific diagnostic group can see useful applications in other areas because of the type of cognitive and functional problem supported.

Conceptualizing ATC in terms of cognitive function (such as alerting, distracting, prompting, navigating, reminding, and storing and displaying; see Gillespie *et al.*, 2012) provides a coherent and, most importantly, useful framework. First, this conceptualization facilitates prescription, because neuropsychological tests can be mapped onto the cognitive functions and thus be used to indicate suitable ATC. Second, this conceptualization enables generalizing results from trials of specific ATC devices toward general ATC functions.

In addition, conceptualizing ATC in terms of cognitive function enables us to identify gaps. For example, 63 percent of the reviewed studies reported reminding and prompting interventions. While these had the greatest amount of current evidence for their use, the preponderance of these devices should not obscure the potential of ATC to support additional cognitive functions. There is increasing evidence for the efficacy of ATC to support attention, emotion regulation, experience of self in relation to place, and memory. The development of computer systems that closely emulate the cognitive functions of object, face, and voice recognition, object tracking, perception of facial emotion, lexical and word comprehension, semantic search, and complex problem solution, promise many more areas of cognitive support in the near future, but these potentials can only come to fruition if the technology can overcome the challenges identified in the present chapter.

We expect the coming decades to bring even greater innovations. The maturation of artificial intelligence, speech recognition, object recognition, sensor technologies, and mobile computing will likely coalesce in assistive technologies for cognition that are both innovative and powerful. We do hope that some of these innovations will surprise (in a good way), thus rendering our predictions about the potentials and challenges of ATC dated, maybe even amusing. However, we hope too that the idea of conceptualizing ATC in terms of cognitive function, within the neuro-socio-technical model, will better survive the test of time. The field of ATC will always entail coordination between brain processes, technology, and the social world. Our authors have provided us with the state of the science, from which we look forward to technological developments that take their inspiration from cognition. The technologies supporting the cognitive functions will change, but the needs of those with brain impairments will continue to be the necessities that act as mothers to invention.

References

Ajzen, I. (1991). The Theory of Planned Behavior. *Organizational Behavior and Human Decision Processes*, 50: 179–211.

Ajzen, I. and Fishbein, M. (1980). *Understanding Attitudes and Predicting Social Behavior.* Englewood Cliffs, NJ: Prentice-Hall.

Alloway, T. P. and Alloway, R. G. (2010). Investigating the Predictive Roles of Working Memory and IQ in Academic Attainment. *Journal of Experimental Child Psychology*, 106: 20–9.

Baltes, P. B. (1997). On the Incomplete Architecture of Human Ontogeny. Selection, Optimization and Compensation as Foundation of Developmental Theory. *The American Psychologist*, 52(4): 366–80.

Bateson, G. (1972). *Steps to an Ecology of Mind.* New York, NY: Ballantine Books.

Bauer, M. (2014). *Atoms, Bytes and Genes: Public Resistance and Socio-technical Responses.* London, UK: Routledge.

Bechara, A., Damasio, H., Tranel, D., and Damasio, A. R. (1997). Deciding Advantageously before Knowing the Advantageous Strategy. *Science*, 275(5304): 1293–5.

Best, C., O'Neill, B., and Gillespie, A. (2013). Assistive Technology for Cognition: Enabling Activities of Daily Living. In M. M. Cruz-Cunha, I. M. Miranda, and P. Goncalves (eds), *Handbook of Research on ICTs for Human-Centered Healthcare and Social Care Services*. Hershey, PA: IGI Global.

Best, C., O'Neill, B., and Gillespie, A. (2014). Assistive Technology for Cognition: An Updated Review. In G. Naik and Y. Guo (eds), *Emerging Theory and Practice in Neuroprosthetics*. Hershey, PA: IGI Global.

Boger, J., Dunal, L., Quraishi, M., and Turcotte, N. (2014). The Identification of Assistive Technologies Being Used to Support the Daily Occupations of Community-Dwelling Older Adults With Dementia: A Cross-Sectional Pilot Study. *Disability and Rehabilitation: Assistive Technology*, 9(1): 17–30.

Bond, M. R., Brooks, D. N., and McKinlay, W. (1979). Burdens Imposed on the Relatives of Those with Severe Brain Damage due to Injury. *Acta Neurochirurgia Supplement*, 28: 124–5.

Bowen, C., Yeates, G., and Palmer, S. (2010). *A Relational Approach to Rehabilitation: Thinking about Relationships after Brain Injury*. London, UK: Karnac Books.

Burgess, P. W., Gonen-Yaacovi, G., and Volle, E. (2011). Functional Neuroimaging Studies of Prospective Memory: What Have we Learnt so far? *Neuropsychologia*, 49(8): 2246–57.

Carr, N. (2010). *The Shallows: How the Internet is Changing the Way we Think, Read and Remember*. London, UK: Atlantic Books Ltd.

Ericsson, K. A. and Simon, H. A. (1993). *Protocol Analysis: Verbal Reports as Data*. Cambridge, MA: MIT Press.

Fishbein, M. and Ajzen, I. (1975). *Belief, Attitude, Intention and Behavior: An Introduction to Theory and Research*. Reading, MA: Addison-Wesley.

Fleminger, S., Greenwood, R. J., and Oliver, D. L. (2006). Pharmacological Management for Agitation and Aggression in People with Acquired Brain Injury. *Cochrane Database of Systematic Reviews*, 18(4): CD003299.

Gilbert, D. T., Pinel, E. C., Wilson, T. D., Blumberg, S. J., and Wheatley, T. P. (1998). Immune Neglect: A Source of Durability Bias in Affective Forecasting. *Journal of Personality and Social Psychology*, 75(3): 617.

Gillespie, A., Murphy, J., and Place, M. (2010). Divergences of Perspective Between People with Aphasia and their Family Caregivers. *Aphasiology*, 24(12): 1559–75.

Gillespie, A., Best, C., and O'Neill, B. (2012). Cognitive Function and Assistive Technology for Cognition: A Systematic Review. *Journal of the International Neuropsychological Society*, 18(01): 1–19.

Goffman, E. (1963). *Stigma: Notes on the Management of Spoiled Identity*. New York, NY: Touchstone.

Gosling, J. and Oddy, M. (1999). Rearranged Marriages: Marital Relationships After Head Injury. *Brain injury*, 13(10): 785–96.

Heim, M. (1999). *Electric Language: A Philosophical Study of Word Processing*. New Haven, CT: Yale University Press.

Hochberg, L. R., Bacher, D., Jarosiewicz, B., Masse, N. Y., Simeral, J. D., Vogel, J., and Donoghue, J. P. (2012). Reach and Grasp by People with Tetraplegia using a Neurally Controlled Robotic Arm. *Nature*, 485(7398): 372–5.

Hutchins, E. (1995). *Cognition in the Wild*. Cambridge, MA: The MIT Press.

Karniol, R. and Ross, M. (1996). The Motivational Impact of Temporal Focus: Thinking about the Future and the Past. *Annual Review of Psychology*, 47(1): 593–620.

Merton, R. K. (1936). The Unanticipated Consequences of Purposive Social Action. *American Sociological Review*, 1(6): 894–904.

Mihailidis, A., Boger, J., Hoey, J., and Jiancaro, T. (2011). *Zero Effort Technologies: Considerations, Challenges and Use in Health, Wellness and Rehabilitation*. Toronto, Canada: Morgan & Claypool Publishers.

Norman, D. A. (2002). *The Design of Everyday Things*. London, UK: Basic Books.

Oddy, M. and da Silva Ramos, S. (2013). The Clinical and Cost-Benefits of Investing in Neurobehavioural Rehabilitation: A Multi-Centre Study. *Brain Injury*, 27(13–14): 1500–7.

O'Neill, B. and Gillespie, A. (2008). Simulating Naturalistic Instruction: The Case for a Voice Mediated Interface for Assistive Technology for Cognition. *Journal of Assistive Technologies*, 2(2): 22–31.

O'Neill, B., Gillespie, A., and Moran, K. (2010). Scaffolding Rehabilitation Behaviour using a Voice Mediated Assistive Technology for Cognition. *Neuropsychological Rehabilitation*, 18: 1–19.

Orpwood, R., Sixsmith, A., Torrington, J., Chadd, J., Gibson, G., and Chalfont, G. (2007). Designing Technology to Support Quality of Life of People with Dementia. *Technology and Disability*, 19: 103–12.

Pea, R. D. (2004). The Social and Technological Dimensions of Scaffolding and Related Theoretical Concepts for Learning, Education and Human Activity. *The Journal of the Learning Sciences*, 13(3): 423–51.

Pirsiavash, H. and Ramanan, D. (2012). Detecting Activities of Daily Living in First-Person Camera Views. In *Computer Vision and Pattern Recognition (CVPR), 2012 IEEE Conference* (pp. 2847–54).

Ring, D. H. (1947). *Mobile Telephony – Wide Area Coverage – Case 20564*. Bell Telephone Laboratories. December 11, 1947. Available at: www.privateline.com/archive/Ringcellreport1947.pdf (accessed 23 June 2014).

Schacter, D. L., Addis, D. R., and Buckner, R. L. (2008). Episodic Simulation of Future Events. *Annals of the New York Academy of Sciences*, 1124(1): 39–60.

Taleb, N. N. (2010). *The Black Swan: The Impact of the Highly Improbable Fragility*. London, UK: Random House.

Tomasello, M., Carpenter, M., Call, J., Behne, T., and Moll, H. (2005). Understanding and Sharing Intentions: The Origins of Cultural Cognition. *Behavioral and Brain Sciences*, 28(05): 675–91.

Vygotsky, L. S. (1997). *The Collected Works of L. S. Vygotsky* (Vol. 4, edited by R. W. Rieber). New York: Plenum Press.

Wagoner, B. and Gillespie, A. (2014). Sociocultural Mediators of Remembering: An Extension of Bartlett's Method of Repeated Reproduction. *British Journal of Social Psychology*. doi: 10.1111/bjso.12059.

Weinstein, N. D. (1982). Unrealistic Optimism about Susceptibility to Health Problems. *Journal of Behavioral Medicine*, 5(4): 441–60.

Wherton, J. P. and Monk, A. F. (2008). Technological Opportunities for Supporting People with Dementia who are Living at Home. *International Journal of Human-Computer Studies*, 66(8): 571–86.

Wilson, B. A., Emslie, H. C., Quirk, K., and Evans, J. J. (2001). Reducing Everyday Memory and Planning Problems by Means of a Paging System: A Randomised Control Crossover Study. *Journal of Neurology, Neurosurgery and Psychiatry*, 70: 477–82.

Wood, R. L. (2001). Understanding Neurobehavioural Disability. In R. L. Wood and T. M. McMillan (eds), *Neurobehavioural Disability and Social Handicap Following Traumatic Brain Injury*. Hove, UK: Psychology Press.

World Health Organization. (2002). *Towards a Common Language for Functioning, Disability and Health* (ICF). Geneva. Available at: www.who.int/classifications/icf/site/beginners/bg.pdf (accessed 17 May 2013).

Worthington, A. D., Matthews, S., Melia, Y., and Oddy, M. (2006). Cost-benefits Associated with Social Outcome from Neurobehavioural Rehabilitation. *Brain Injury*, 20(9): 947–57.

AUTHOR INDEX

SUBJECT INDEX